THE 4:3 INTERMITTENT FASTING DIET COOKBOOK

A Simple Guide to Losing Weight Quickly, Lowering Cholesterol, Boosting Autophagy, and Improving Metabolic Health

Dr. Anna Fennell

COPYRIGHT

TABLE OF CONTENTS

INTRODUCTION

The 4 3 Diet is designed around a simple yet highly effective weekly cycle aimed at promoting both nutritional balance and intermittent fasting benefits. This diet consists of four days where individuals follow a regular, balanced eating plan, allowing them to enjoy a wide variety of foods without stringent restrictions. These four days are followed by three days of controlled fasting, where calorie intake is significantly reduced in a structured manner.

This cycle repeats every week, creating a rhythmic pattern that integrates seamlessly into everyday life. The key principle behind the 4 3 Diet is to develop a manageable and sustainable eating routine that can be adhered to over the long term. Unlike many other diets that require extreme dietary restrictions or constant vigilance, the 4 3 Diet offers a more flexible and less demanding approach. It aims to reduce the stress and difficulty often associated with dieting, making it easier for individuals to maintain their commitment and achieve their health and weight management goals.

By allowing for periods of normal eating, participants can satisfy their nutritional needs and enjoy their favorite foods, which helps in reducing feelings of deprivation and maintaining motivation. On the controlled fasting days, the diet taps into the benefits of intermittent fasting, such as improved metabolic health and enhanced weight loss. This balanced approach ensures that individuals do not feel overwhelmed or burnt out, which is a common issue with more restrictive dieting methods.

Ultimately, the 4 3 Diet promotes a balanced lifestyle that supports both physical and mental well-being. Its cyclical nature ensures that individuals can enjoy their meals while still making significant progress towards their health objectives. This makes the 4 3 Diet not only a practical choice but also a sustainable one for long-term success.

CHAPTER ONE

WHAT PRECISELY IS 4 3 DIET?

The 4 3 Diet is a specific type of intermittent fasting regimen designed to balance periods of regular eating with intervals of controlled fasting over the course of a week. This diet plan operates on a cycle, beginning with four days where individuals consume regular, balanced meals. During these four days, the focus is on eating nutritious foods that provide a well-rounded diet, ensuring all necessary vitamins and minerals are included.

After these initial four days of normal eating, the cycle transitions into a phase of controlled fasting for the next three days. During these fasting days, the caloric intake is significantly reduced, but it is not a complete fast. Instead, individuals consume a limited number of calories, often focusing on foods that are low in calories but still provide essential nutrients to maintain energy levels and health.

The idea behind this diet is to create a sustainable pattern of eating and fasting that can be maintained over the long term, potentially leading to benefits such as weight loss, improved metabolic health, and better regulation of blood sugar levels. Here's a detailed breakdown of how the 4 3 Diet works and what you can expect during each phase of the cycle.

The Philosophy of the 4:3 Diet

The philosophy underpinning the 4:3 Diet revolves around the concept of intermittent fasting as a means to promote health and well-being. This dietary approach acknowledges the body's ability to adapt to periods of both nourishment and abstention, leveraging this natural rhythm to support metabolic function and overall health.

At its core, the 4:3 Diet emphasizes balance and moderation, advocating for a structured approach to eating that alternates between periods of regular, balanced nutrition and controlled fasting. By incorporating this cyclical pattern into one's eating habits, proponents of the 4:3 Diet believe it can lead to various health benefits, including weight management, improved insulin sensitivity, and metabolic flexibility.

The philosophy behind the 4:3 Diet encourages individuals to view fasting not as deprivation, but as an opportunity for the body to reset and rejuvenate. By allowing the digestive system a break from constant processing, fasting periods are thought to promote cellular repair, autophagy (the body's natural process of cleaning out damaged cells), and hormonal balance.

Moreover, the 4:3 Diet promotes mindfulness and awareness around food choices, encouraging individuals to prioritize nutrient-dense foods during eating periods and to listen to their body's hunger and satiety cues. This mindful approach to eating can foster a healthier relationship with food and support long-term dietary adherence.

Overall, the philosophy of the 4:3 Diet embraces the idea of harnessing the body's innate ability to adapt to varying conditions, promoting health and vitality through a balanced integration of nourishment and occasional fasting.

Cultivating Awareness Around Food Choices

Cultivating awareness around food choices involves developing a mindful approach to eating that prioritizes conscious decision-making and understanding the impact of food on both physical and mental well-being. This process encompasses several key aspects:

1. Mindful Eating Practices: Practicing mindfulness while eating involves paying full attention to the sensory experience of eating, including the taste, texture, and aroma of food. This approach encourages individuals to slow down, savor each bite, and fully appreciate the nourishment their food provides.

2. Understanding Nutritional Content: Developing awareness of the nutritional content of different foods enables individuals to make informed choices that support their health goals. This includes recognizing the macronutrient (carbohydrates,

proteins, fats) and micronutrient (vitamins, minerals) profiles of foods and how they contribute to overall nutrition.

3. Listening to Hunger and Satiety Cues: Tuning in to the body's hunger and satiety signals is crucial for maintaining a healthy relationship with food. Cultivating awareness of these cues helps individuals distinguish between physical hunger and emotional or environmental triggers for eating, allowing for more intuitive eating patterns.

4. Considering Food Origins and Sustainability: Being mindful of where food comes from and its environmental impact can influence food choices. This includes supporting local and sustainable food

sources, reducing food waste, and considering the ethical implications of food production practices.

5. Practicing Moderation and Balance: Cultivating awareness around food choices involves finding a balance between enjoying indulgent foods in moderation and prioritizing nutrient-dense options that support overall health. This approach encourages flexibility and avoids rigid dietary rules that may lead to feelings of deprivation or guilt.

6. Reflecting on Personal Values and Goals: Taking time to reflect on personal values and health goals can guide food choices aligned with individual priorities. This may involve considering factors

such as cultural traditions, ethical beliefs, and specific dietary preferences or restrictions.

By cultivating awareness around food choices, individuals can develop a more intentional and empowered relationship with food, promoting both physical health and emotional well-being.

CHAPTER TWO

THE MENTAL AND EMOTIONAL ADVANTAGES OF FASTING

The mental and emotional benefits of fasting are multifaceted, encompassing improvements in cognitive function, emotional regulation, and overall mental clarity. Here's an exploration of these benefits:

1. Enhanced Cognitive Function: Fasting has been shown to improve various aspects of brain function, including memory, focus, and mental clarity. The reduction in blood glucose levels during fasting can lead to increased production of brain-derived

neurotrophic factor (BDNF), a protein that supports the growth and maintenance of neurons. This can enhance learning and memory while also protecting against neurodegenerative diseases.

2. Improved Emotional Regulation: Fasting can help regulate mood and emotional responses. By stabilizing blood sugar levels and reducing inflammation, fasting can minimize mood swings and improve emotional stability. This helps individuals manage stress and anxiety more effectively.

3. Increased Mental Clarity and Focus: Many people report experiencing heightened mental clarity and focus during fasting periods. Without the constant

need to digest food, the body can allocate more energy towards cognitive processes. This can lead to a sharper mind and improved problem-solving abilities.

4. Stress Reduction: Fasting can trigger a relaxation response in the body, reducing the levels of cortisol, the stress hormone. Lower cortisol levels can help decrease feelings of stress and anxiety, leading to a calmer and more balanced mental state.

5. Emotional Resilience: The discipline required to adhere to a fasting regimen can build emotional resilience and a sense of accomplishment. Successfully managing the challenges of fasting can

enhance self-control and self-discipline, boosting self-esteem and confidence.

6. Mindfulness and Awareness: Fasting encourages mindfulness and greater awareness of one's body and eating habits. By removing the constant focus on food, individuals can develop a deeper understanding of their hunger cues, emotional triggers, and eating patterns. This can lead to a more mindful and intentional approach to eating, contributing to better mental and emotional health.

7. Spiritual and Reflective Benefits: For many, fasting is not just a physical practice but also a spiritual one. It can provide an opportunity for

introspection, meditation, and spiritual growth. This reflective period can help individuals gain perspective, set personal goals, and find deeper meaning in their daily lives.

In summary, fasting offers numerous mental and emotional benefits that go beyond physical health. By enhancing cognitive function, improving emotional regulation, and fostering mindfulness, fasting can contribute to a more balanced, resilient, and reflective mental state.

Fasting as a Practice of Discipline and Resilience

Fasting as a practice of discipline and resilience involves more than just abstaining from food; it is a holistic approach to self-control and personal growth. Here's an exploration of how fasting fosters these qualities:

1. Building Self-Discipline: Fasting requires a conscious decision to refrain from eating for a set period, which demands a significant amount of self-control and commitment. This practice helps individuals develop the ability to stick to their goals despite temptations, strengthening their overall discipline. The structured nature of fasting schedules reinforces the importance of routine and consistency.

2. Enhancing Willpower: Regularly engaging in fasting can increase one's willpower. By repeatedly facing and overcoming the urge to eat, individuals

can build their capacity to resist other temptations and distractions in various areas of life. This enhanced willpower can translate into better decision-making and greater control over impulsive behaviors.

3. Fostering Resilience: Fasting can be challenging, especially during the initial stages when the body is adjusting to a new eating pattern. Overcoming these challenges can foster resilience, teaching individuals to endure discomfort and delay gratification. This ability to withstand temporary hardships builds mental and emotional strength, making it easier to cope with other stressors and difficulties.

4. Cultivating Patience and Persistence: The practice of fasting requires patience, as the benefits often manifest gradually over time. This patience, coupled with the persistence needed to adhere to fasting schedules, helps individuals develop a long-term perspective on achieving their goals. It encourages a mindset that values consistent effort and dedication.

5. Enhancing Emotional Control: Fasting can lead to greater emotional regulation by teaching individuals to manage feelings of hunger and the emotions associated with it, such as irritability or frustration. This control over emotional responses can extend to other areas of life, helping individuals maintain composure and react more thoughtfully in stressful situations.

6. Developing a Sense of Achievement: Successfully completing fasting periods provides a sense of accomplishment. This achievement can boost self-esteem and confidence, reinforcing the belief in one's ability to set and meet challenging goals. Celebrating these successes, no matter how small, can motivate individuals to pursue further self-improvement.

7. Encouraging Reflective Practices: The introspective nature of fasting often leads individuals to reflect on their habits, motivations, and personal growth. This period of reflection can provide valuable insights into one's strengths and areas for improvement, fostering a deeper understanding of oneself.

In summary, fasting as a practice of discipline and resilience goes beyond physical benefits. It cultivates self-discipline, enhances willpower, fosters resilience, and promotes emotional control. By encouraging patience, persistence, and reflection, fasting helps individuals develop a stronger, more resilient mindset that can positively impact various aspects of their lives.

Exploring the Psychological Effects of Intermittent Fasting

Exploring the psychological effects of intermittent fasting reveals a range of mental and emotional benefits that extend beyond physical health improvements. Here are some key psychological effects associated with intermittent fasting:

1. Improved Cognitive Function: Intermittent fasting has been shown to enhance various aspects of brain function, including memory, learning, and overall cognitive performance. This is partly due to increased production of brain-derived neurotrophic factor (BDNF), a protein that supports neuron growth and maintenance, which can lead to sharper mental acuity and better cognitive health.

2. Enhanced Mood and Emotional Stability: By stabilizing blood sugar levels and reducing inflammation, intermittent fasting can help improve mood and reduce the risk of mood swings. Many individuals report feeling more emotionally

balanced and less prone to anxiety and depression during fasting periods.

3. Increased Mental Clarity and Focus: Many people experience heightened mental clarity and focus during fasting periods. Without the constant need to digest food, the body can allocate more energy to cognitive processes, leading to improved concentration and productivity.

4. Stress Reduction and Relaxation: Intermittent fasting can reduce levels of cortisol, the body's primary stress hormone. Lower cortisol levels can lead to a reduction in stress and anxiety, promoting a calmer, more relaxed state of mind.

5. Development of Self-Control and Discipline: The practice of intermittent fasting requires a significant amount of self-control and discipline. Successfully adhering to a fasting regimen can strengthen willpower and self-regulation, fostering a greater sense of personal achievement and confidence.

6. Mindfulness and Enhanced Awareness: Fasting encourages mindfulness and greater awareness of eating habits and hunger cues. This heightened awareness can lead to more mindful eating practices, where individuals become more attuned to their body's needs and more deliberate in their food choices.

7. Increased Emotional Resilience: The challenges of intermittent fasting can build emotional resilience. By enduring and overcoming the discomfort of hunger, individuals can develop greater emotional strength and the ability to cope with other stressors and difficulties in life.

8. Spiritual and Reflective Benefits: For many, intermittent fasting is not just a dietary practice but also a time for introspection and spiritual growth. Fasting periods can provide an opportunity for meditation, reflection, and personal growth, helping individuals gain new perspectives and set meaningful goals.

9. Enhanced Sense of Achievement and Self-Esteem: Successfully completing fasting periods can provide a significant sense of accomplishment. This boost in self-esteem and confidence can motivate individuals to pursue further personal development and set and achieve other challenging goals.

In summary, the psychological effects of intermittent fasting encompass improvements in cognitive function, mood stability, mental clarity, and stress reduction. It also fosters self-discipline, mindfulness, emotional resilience, and personal growth. These benefits contribute to a more balanced and empowered mental and emotional state, enhancing overall well-being.

CHAPTER THREE

NOURISHING THE BODY, MIND, AND SPIRIT

Nourishing the body, mind, and spirit involves a holistic approach to health and well-being that encompasses physical nutrition, mental stimulation, and spiritual growth. Here's an exploration of how to achieve this comprehensive nourishment:

Nourishing the Body

1. Balanced Diet: Consuming a variety of nutrient-dense foods is essential for maintaining physical health. This includes a balanced intake of fruits, vegetables, whole grains, lean proteins, and healthy fats. Each food group provides vital nutrients that support bodily functions, energy levels, and overall health.

2. Hydration: Drinking adequate water throughout the day is crucial for maintaining bodily functions, including digestion, circulation, and temperature regulation. Proper hydration also supports cognitive function and energy levels.

3. Regular Physical Activity: Engaging in regular exercise, whether it's aerobic activities, strength

training, or flexibility exercises, helps maintain a healthy weight, improves cardiovascular health, and enhances overall physical fitness. Exercise also releases endorphins, which can boost mood and reduce stress.

4. Rest and Recovery: Ensuring adequate sleep and rest is vital for physical health. Sleep allows the body to repair and rejuvenate, supporting immune function, memory, and cognitive performance. Rest days between intense physical activities also help prevent injury and promote muscle recovery.

Nourishing the Mind

1. Continuous Learning: Engaging in activities that stimulate the mind, such as reading, solving puzzles, or learning new skills, helps maintain cognitive function and promotes lifelong learning. This mental stimulation can improve memory, focus, and problem-solving abilities.

2. Mindfulness and Meditation: Practicing mindfulness and meditation can enhance mental clarity, reduce stress, and improve emotional regulation. These practices encourage living in the present moment and can help manage anxiety and depressive symptoms.

3. Creative Expression: Participating in creative activities like art, music, writing, or dance can

provide a mental outlet for self-expression and stress relief. Creative expression fosters innovation and can be a powerful tool for emotional healing and personal growth.

4. Social Connections: Building and maintaining healthy relationships with family, friends, and community members is crucial for mental well-being. Social interactions provide emotional support, reduce feelings of loneliness, and enhance a sense of belonging.

Nourishing the Spirit

1. Spiritual Practices: Engaging in spiritual practices, such as prayer, meditation, or attending religious services, can provide a sense of purpose and connection to something greater than oneself. These practices can offer comfort, guidance, and a sense of peace.

2. Reflection and Gratitude: Taking time for self-reflection and practicing gratitude can enhance spiritual well-being. Reflecting on personal experiences and expressing gratitude for life's blessings can foster a positive outlook and deepen one's spiritual awareness.

3. Connection with Nature: Spending time in nature can be a rejuvenating experience for the spirit.

Activities like walking in the park, hiking, or simply sitting in a garden can promote a sense of tranquility and connection to the natural world.

4. Acts of Kindness and Service: Engaging in acts of kindness and service to others can nourish the spirit by fostering a sense of compassion and altruism. Helping others can create a sense of fulfillment and strengthen community bonds.

Incorporating Mind-Body Practices into Your Fasting Routine

Incorporating mind-body practices into your fasting routine can enhance your overall fasting experience and promote holistic well-being. Here are some ways to integrate these practices into your fasting regimen:

1. Mindful Eating: During your eating windows, practice mindful eating by paying full attention to the sensory experience of eating. Chew your food slowly, savoring each bite, and fully experiencing the flavors and textures. This can help you feel more satisfied with your meals and prevent overeating.

2. Mindfulness Meditation: Dedicate time each day to mindfulness meditation, either before or after your fasting periods. Sit quietly and focus on your breath or use guided meditation exercises to cultivate present-moment awareness. Mindfulness meditation can help reduce stress, increase self-awareness, and improve emotional regulation.

3. Yoga and Stretching: Incorporate gentle yoga or stretching exercises into your fasting routine to promote physical relaxation and flexibility. Practice gentle poses that focus on deep breathing and gentle movements to help release tension and improve circulation. Yoga can also help calm the mind and promote a sense of inner peace.

4. Breathing Exercises: Practice deep breathing exercises, such as diaphragmatic breathing or alternate nostril breathing, to help relax the body and reduce stress levels. Deep breathing can help activate the parasympathetic nervous system, promoting a state of relaxation and calmness.

5. Visualization Techniques: Use visualization techniques to focus your mind and enhance your fasting experience. Visualize yourself achieving your health goals, feeling energized and vibrant, or overcoming any challenges you may encounter during fasting. Visualization can help reinforce positive beliefs and intentions, enhancing your motivation and determination.

6. Journaling: Keep a fasting journal to track your progress, reflect on your experiences, and explore your thoughts and feelings related to fasting. Use your journal as a tool for self-reflection and self-discovery, noting any insights or observations that arise during your fasting journey.

7. Nature Walks: Take regular walks in nature during your fasting periods to connect with the natural world and promote a sense of grounding and tranquility. Spend time in green spaces, such as parks or forests, and immerse yourself in the sights, sounds, and smells of nature. Nature walks can help reduce stress, boost mood, and enhance overall well-being.

Incorporating these mind-body practices into your fasting routine can help you cultivate a deeper sense of awareness, relaxation, and resilience, supporting your overall health and well-being during fasting periods.v

Creating Rituals Around Food and Fasting

Creating rituals around food and fasting can add meaning, structure, and mindfulness to your eating habits and fasting routine. Here are some ways to incorporate rituals into your approach to food and fasting:

Meal Preparation: Dedicate time to preparing your meals mindfully, focusing on selecting fresh, nourishing ingredients and engaging in the cooking process with intention and care. Consider incorporating soothing music, aromatherapy, or gratitude practices into your meal preparation routine to enhance the experience.

Setting the Table: Create a tranquil and inviting space for your meals by setting the table with intention. Use beautiful tableware, light candles, or arrange fresh flowers to elevate the ambiance and create a sense of occasion around your eating rituals.

Mindful Eating Practices: Slow down and savor each bite of your meals by practicing mindful eating. Pay attention to the flavors, textures, and sensations of the food, and chew slowly to fully experience the nourishment it provides. Avoid distractions like screens or multitasking during meals to focus your attention on the present moment.

Fasting Rituals: Establish rituals to mark the beginning and end of fasting periods. This could involve setting an intention or reflection at the start of each fast, and expressing gratitude or celebrating your accomplishment at the end. Consider incorporating practices like meditation, journaling, or gentle movement to support you during fasting periods.

Daily Reflection: Take time each day to reflect on your eating habits and fasting experience. Journaling about your thoughts, feelings, and observations can help deepen your awareness and understanding of your relationship with food and fasting. Use this reflection time to set intentions, identify areas for growth, and celebrate your successes.

Connection with Nature: Incorporate rituals that connect you with nature and the natural rhythms of the earth. Take walks outdoors, practice grounding exercises like barefoot walking or gardening, or simply spend time in nature to cultivate a sense of balance and harmony with the world around you.

Community and Sharing: Share your food rituals and fasting experiences with loved ones or like-minded individuals in your community. Consider hosting shared meals, potlucks, or fasting support groups to create a sense of connection and camaraderie around your dietary practices.

Gratitude Practices: Cultivate gratitude for the food you eat and the nourishment it provides by incorporating gratitude practices into your eating rituals. Take a moment before each meal to express thanks for the abundance of food, the hands that prepared it, and the opportunity to nourish your body and soul.

By creating meaningful rituals around food and fasting, you can enhance your awareness, appreciation, and enjoyment of the eating experience while supporting your overall health and well-being.

CHAPTER FOUR

FASTING SERVES AS A TRIGGER FOR SELF-EXPLORATION

Fasting as a catalyst for self-discovery offers a unique opportunity to explore and understand various aspects of oneself, fostering personal growth and self-awareness. Here are several ways in which fasting can lead to self-discovery:

Enhanced Self-Awareness

1. Mindful Observation: During fasting, you become more attuned to your body's signals and needs. This heightened awareness can help you identify patterns and triggers related to hunger, emotions, and cravings, providing valuable insights into your eating habits and emotional responses.

2. Emotional Insight: Fasting can bring emotions to the surface, allowing you to recognize and address underlying feelings that may have been masked by habitual eating. By confronting these emotions, you can develop a deeper understanding of your emotional landscape and learn healthier ways to cope.

Mental Clarity and Focus

1. Improved Concentration: Many people report increased mental clarity and focus during fasting periods. This enhanced cognitive function can provide the mental space needed to reflect on your life, set goals, and gain new perspectives on personal challenges.

2. Reflective Practices: Use the mental clarity gained from fasting to engage in reflective practices such as journaling, meditation, or contemplation. These activities can help you process thoughts and experiences, leading to greater self-awareness and personal insights.

Spiritual Growth

1. Spiritual Reflection: Fasting has been used for centuries as a spiritual practice in many cultures. It can be a time for spiritual reflection, prayer, and connection to a higher purpose. This spiritual engagement can lead to profound self-discovery and a deeper sense of meaning and purpose in life.

2. Mind-Body Connection: Fasting emphasizes the connection between the mind and body, encouraging you to listen to and honor both. This holistic awareness can foster a sense of unity and balance, promoting overall well-being and spiritual growth.

Developing Discipline and Resilience

1. Building Willpower: The discipline required to adhere to a fasting regimen strengthens willpower and self-control. This practice can enhance your ability to set and achieve goals, manage impulses, and maintain commitments in other areas of life.

2. Overcoming Challenges: Fasting presents physical and mental challenges that test your resilience. Overcoming these challenges can build inner strength, boost confidence, and reveal your capacity to endure and thrive despite difficulties.

Personal Growth and Transformation

1. Breaking Habits: Fasting can help you break free from unhealthy eating patterns and habits. By stepping back from routine behaviors, you can reassess and realign your lifestyle choices with your health and wellness goals.

2. Setting Intentions: Use fasting as a time to set intentions for personal growth and transformation. Whether it's adopting healthier habits, pursuing new interests, or letting go of what no longer serves you, fasting can be a powerful catalyst for positive change.

Cultivating Gratitude and Appreciation

1. Appreciation for Food: Fasting can deepen your appreciation for food and nourishment. The absence of food can make you more grateful for the sustenance it provides, fostering a healthier relationship with eating and an appreciation for the abundance in your life.

2. Gratitude Practices: Incorporate gratitude practices into your fasting routine. Reflect on the things you are grateful for, both big and small, to cultivate a positive outlook and enhance your overall sense of well-being.

Setting Intentions and Goals Beyond Weight Loss

Setting intentions and goals beyond weight loss when fasting can provide deeper, more meaningful motivations that foster overall well-being. Here are some ways to establish such intentions and goals:

Enhancing Physical Health

1. Improving Metabolic Health: Focus on goals like stabilizing blood sugar levels, improving cholesterol profiles, and reducing inflammation. Regular fasting can support metabolic health, helping to prevent chronic diseases like diabetes and heart disease.

2. Boosting Energy Levels: Aim to enhance your energy and vitality. By giving your digestive system a break and promoting cellular repair, fasting can increase your overall energy levels and make you feel more vibrant.

3. Promoting Longevity: Set intentions to support longevity and healthy aging. Fasting can stimulate autophagy, the body's way of cleaning out damaged cells, which may contribute to a longer, healthier life.

Mental and Emotional Well-Being

1. Reducing Stress and Anxiety: Use fasting periods to develop better stress management techniques. Engage in mindfulness practices, meditation, or yoga to cultivate a calm and centered mind.

2. Enhancing Mental Clarity: Set goals to improve mental clarity and cognitive function. Many find that fasting helps clear the mind and enhance focus, which can be beneficial for work, study, or personal projects.

3. Developing Emotional Resilience: Aim to build emotional resilience by observing how fasting affects your moods and emotional responses. Use

this time to develop healthier coping mechanisms and emotional regulation strategies.

Spiritual Growth

1. Deepening Spiritual Practice: Incorporate spiritual practices such as prayer, meditation, or contemplation into your fasting routine. Set intentions to deepen your spiritual understanding and connection.

2. Cultivating Inner Peace: Use fasting as a time to seek inner peace and tranquility. Focus on practices

that help you feel centered and balanced, fostering a sense of harmony and inner calm.

Building Discipline and Personal Growth

1. Strengthening Willpower: Use fasting as a tool to build willpower and self-discipline. The act of fasting itself can be a powerful exercise in self-control and determination, which can translate into other areas of life.

2. Overcoming Challenges: Set goals to overcome personal challenges and limitations. Fasting can teach perseverance and resilience, showing you that

you are capable of more than you may have realized.

Cultivating Gratitude and Mindfulness

1. Appreciating Nourishment: Develop a deeper appreciation for food and nourishment. Use fasting periods to reflect on the value of food, the effort it takes to prepare it, and the pleasure of eating mindfully.

2. Living in the Present: Set intentions to live more fully in the present moment. Use fasting as a

practice of mindfulness, paying attention to your body's signals and the experience of eating.

Enhancing Relationships

1. Fostering Connection: Use fasting as an opportunity to connect with others who are also exploring fasting or similar practices. Share your experiences, support each other, and build a sense of community.

2. Improving Communication: Set goals to improve your communication and relationships. The clarity and mindfulness that can come from fasting may

help you to be more present and attentive in your interactions with others.

Supporting Ethical and Environmental Goals

1. Practicing Sustainability: Reflect on your food choices and their impact on the environment. Use fasting as a time to consider more sustainable and ethical eating habits, such as reducing food waste or choosing plant-based options.

2. Aligning with Values: Set intentions that align with your personal values. This might include

supporting local farmers, choosing organic produce, or reducing your carbon footprint.

Embracing Change and Embodying Resilience

Embracing change and embodying resilience are crucial aspects of personal growth and well-being. Here are some ways to integrate these principles into your life:

Understanding the Nature of Change

1. Accepting Impermanence: Recognize that change is an inherent part of life. Accepting the

impermanent nature of circumstances can help you remain adaptable and open to new experiences.

2. Viewing Change as Opportunity: Instead of fearing change, see it as an opportunity for growth and improvement. Each change, whether positive or negative, can offer valuable lessons and new perspectives.

Cultivating a Resilient Mindset

1. Building Mental Toughness: Strengthen your mental resilience by challenging yourself regularly.

This can be through physical exercise, mental tasks, or stepping out of your comfort zone in small ways.

2. Positive Self-Talk: Practice positive self-talk to build confidence and resilience. Remind yourself of past successes and your ability to overcome challenges.

3. Embracing Failure: View failures as stepping stones rather than setbacks. Each failure provides insights and experiences that contribute to future success.

Developing Healthy Coping Mechanisms

1. Mindfulness and Meditation: Incorporate mindfulness and meditation practices to manage stress and maintain a balanced perspective. These practices can help you stay grounded and present during times of change.

2. Emotional Regulation: Learn techniques to manage your emotions effectively. This could include deep breathing exercises, journaling, or seeking support from friends or professionals.

3. Physical Well-Being: Maintain your physical health through regular exercise, proper nutrition,

and adequate rest. A healthy body supports a resilient mind.

Strengthening Social Connections

1. Building a Support Network: Surround yourself with supportive and positive people. A strong social network provides emotional support, advice, and encouragement during challenging times.

2. Communicating Openly: Practice open and honest communication with those around you. Sharing your experiences and listening to others fosters mutual understanding and support.

Setting Realistic Goals

1. Short-Term Goals: Set achievable short-term goals that lead towards larger aspirations. Celebrating small victories along the way can boost motivation and resilience.

2. Long-Term Vision: Maintain a clear vision of your long-term goals. This vision can provide direction and purpose, helping you stay focused during periods of change.

Embracing Flexibility

1. Adapting to New Situations: Stay flexible and open to adapting your plans and strategies as circumstances change. Flexibility allows you to navigate unexpected challenges more effectively.

2. Continuous Learning: Commit to lifelong learning and self-improvement. Embrace new skills, knowledge, and experiences to remain adaptable and resilient.

Practicing Gratitude

1. Daily Gratitude: Practice daily gratitude by reflecting on the positive aspects of your life. Gratitude can shift your focus from what is lacking to what is abundant, fostering a resilient mindset.

2. Acknowledging Growth: Recognize and celebrate your personal growth and achievements, no matter how small. Acknowledging progress reinforces your resilience and commitment to embracing change.

CHAPTER FIVE

INCORPORATING FASTING INTO YOUR LIFESTYLE

Integrating fasting into your lifestyle can be a transformative approach to improving your overall health and well-being. Here are some strategies and tips to help you seamlessly incorporate fasting into your daily routine:

Understanding the Basics

1. Research Different Fasting Methods: There are various fasting protocols such as intermittent

fasting (e.g., 16:8, 5:2), alternate-day fasting, and extended fasting. Understand each method and choose one that aligns with your lifestyle and health goals.

2. Consult with a Healthcare Professional: Before starting any fasting regimen, especially if you have underlying health conditions or are taking medications, consult with a healthcare provider to ensure it's safe for you.

Planning Your Fasting Schedule

1. Start Gradually: If you're new to fasting, begin with a shorter fasting period and gradually increase the duration as your body adapts. For instance, start with a 12-hour fast and slowly work up to a 16-hour fast.

2. Consistency is Key: Try to stick to a regular fasting schedule. Consistency helps your body get used to the new eating pattern, making it easier to maintain in the long run.

Nutrition During Eating Windows

1. Prioritize Nutrient-Dense Foods: During your eating windows, focus on consuming a balanced diet rich in whole foods, including vegetables, fruits, lean proteins, healthy fats, and whole grains.

2. Stay Hydrated: Drink plenty of water throughout the day, including during fasting periods. Herbal teas and black coffee (without sugar or cream) are also good options that can help you stay hydrated without breaking your fast.

3. Avoid Overeating: It can be tempting to overeat when you break your fast, but try to maintain portion control to avoid digestive discomfort and to ensure you're not consuming more calories than necessary.

Managing Social Situations

1. Communicate Your Plan: Inform friends and family about your fasting routine. This can help you navigate social situations and gatherings more easily and get support from those around you.

2. Plan Ahead: If you have social events that involve food, plan your fasting schedule around these events. You can adjust your eating window to coincide with meal times during these occasions.

Incorporating Physical Activity

1. Exercise Timing: Determine the best time for you to exercise in relation to your fasting schedule. Some people prefer to work out during their fasting window, while others feel more energetic and perform better after eating.

2. Listen to Your Body: Pay attention to how your body responds to exercise while fasting. Adjust the intensity and timing of your workouts based on your energy levels and how you feel.

Monitoring Your Progress

1. Track Your Results: Keep a journal to track your fasting schedule, meals, energy levels, mood, and any changes in weight or health markers. This can help you identify patterns and make necessary adjustments.

2. Be Patient: Results from fasting may take time. Be patient and give your body time to adjust to the new routine. Focus on the overall benefits rather than immediate results.

Addressing Challenges

1. Managing Hunger: Hunger pangs are common, especially when you start fasting. Drink water, distract yourself with activities, and remind yourself that these feelings often pass quickly.

2. Overcoming Plateaus: If you hit a plateau or don't see the desired results, consider varying your fasting schedule, adjusting your diet, or incorporating new physical activities.

Staying Motivated

1. Set Clear Goals: Establish clear, achievable goals for your fasting journey. Whether it's improved

health markers, weight management, or increased mental clarity, having specific goals can keep you motivated.

2. Join a Community: Connect with others who are also practicing fasting. Sharing experiences, tips, and support can help you stay motivated and committed to your fasting lifestyle.

Creating a Sustainable Fasting Routine

Creating a sustainable fasting routine can help you achieve long-term health benefits and make fasting a seamless part of your daily life. Here are some steps to establish and maintain a sustainable fasting routine:

1. Identify Your Goals: Determine why you want to incorporate fasting into your lifestyle. Common goals include weight management, improved metabolic health, increased energy, or enhanced mental clarity. Having clear objectives will help you stay motivated.

2. Assess Your Lifestyle: Consider your daily schedule, work commitments, social activities, and family obligations. Choose a fasting method that fits well with your existing lifestyle to make it easier to adhere to.

Choosing the Right Fasting Method

1. Explore Different Methods: Research various fasting protocols such as intermittent fasting (e.g., 16:8, 5:2), alternate-day fasting, or extended fasting. Select one that aligns with your goals and is manageable for you.

2. Start Small: If you're new to fasting, begin with shorter fasting periods and gradually increase the duration as your body adapts. For example, start with a 12-hour fast and gradually extend it to 16 hours.

Planning Your Fasting and Eating Windows

1. Set a Consistent Schedule: Establish regular fasting and eating windows that fit your routine. Consistency helps your body adjust to the new eating pattern, making it easier to maintain.

2. Align with Your Natural Rhythms: Choose fasting periods that align with your natural body rhythms. For instance, many people find it easier to skip breakfast and eat between noon and 8 PM.

Optimizing Nutrition

1. Prioritize Nutrient-Dense Foods: During your eating windows, focus on a balanced diet rich in whole foods, including vegetables, fruits, lean proteins, healthy fats, and whole grains. Proper nutrition supports your fasting efforts and overall health.

2. Stay Hydrated: Drink plenty of water throughout the day, including during fasting periods. Herbal teas and black coffee (without sugar or cream) are also good options that can help you stay hydrated without breaking your fast.

3. Avoid Overeating: It can be tempting to overeat when breaking your fast, but aim to maintain portion control to avoid digestive discomfort and

ensure you're not consuming more calories than necessary.

Incorporating Physical Activity

1. Find the Best Time to Exercise: Determine when you feel most energetic for physical activity in relation to your fasting schedule. Some people prefer to work out during their fasting window, while others perform better after eating.

2. Listen to Your Body: Pay attention to how your body responds to exercise while fasting. Adjust the

intensity and timing of your workouts based on your energy levels and how you feel.

Managing Challenges

1. Handle Hunger Pangs: Hunger pangs are common, especially when starting. Drink water, distract yourself with activities, and remind yourself that these feelings often pass quickly.

2. Adjust for Social Situations: Plan your fasting schedule around social events involving food. Adjust your eating window to coincide with meal

times during these occasions to maintain your social life while fasting.

3. Overcoming Plateaus: If you hit a plateau or don't see desired results, consider varying your fasting schedule, adjusting your diet, or incorporating new physical activities to stimulate progress.

Staying Motivated

1. Set Clear, Achievable Goals: Establish specific, realistic goals for your fasting journey. Whether it's improving health markers, managing weight, or

increasing mental clarity, having clear goals can keep you motivated.

2. Track Your Progress: Keep a journal to monitor your fasting schedule, meals, energy levels, mood, and any changes in weight or health markers. Tracking progress can help identify patterns and make necessary adjustments.

3. Join a Supportive Community: Connect with others who practice fasting. Sharing experiences, tips, and support can help you stay motivated and committed to your fasting routine.

Embracing the Journey of Holistic Health

Embracing the journey of holistic health involves nurturing every aspect of your well-being, including physical, mental, emotional, and spiritual dimensions. Here's how you can embark on this transformative journey:

Physical Well-Being

1. Nutritious Diet: Focus on consuming whole, nutrient-dense foods that nourish your body. Incorporate plenty of fruits, vegetables, lean proteins, whole grains, and healthy fats into your diet.

2. Regular Exercise: Engage in physical activities that you enjoy, whether it's walking, jogging, yoga, or dancing. Aim for a combination of cardiovascular exercise, strength training, and flexibility exercises.

3. Adequate Rest: Prioritize sleep and establish a consistent sleep schedule. Quality rest is essential for physical recovery, cognitive function, and overall well-being.

Mental and Emotional Wellness

1. Stress Management: Practice stress-reduction techniques such as mindfulness meditation, deep breathing exercises, or progressive muscle relaxation to cultivate inner peace and resilience.

2. Emotional Awareness: Develop self-awareness and emotional intelligence by acknowledging and processing your feelings in a healthy way. Journaling, therapy, or talking to a trusted friend can be helpful in this regard.

3. Positive Mindset: Foster a positive outlook on life by focusing on gratitude, self-compassion, and optimism. Cultivate a habit of reframing negative thoughts into more constructive perspectives.

Spiritual Growth

1. Mindfulness Practice: Cultivate mindfulness through meditation, prayer, or mindful living. Stay present in the moment and connect with your inner self to deepen your spiritual awareness.

2. Connection with Nature: Spend time outdoors, immerse yourself in natural surroundings, and appreciate the beauty and wonder of the world around you. Nature can be a source of inspiration and spiritual rejuvenation.

3. Exploration of Beliefs: Reflect on your values, beliefs, and purpose in life. Engage in spiritual practices or philosophical inquiries that resonate with your innermost truths and aspirations.

Social Connection

1. Supportive Relationships: Cultivate meaningful connections with friends, family, and community members who uplift and support you on your journey to holistic health. Nurture these relationships with care and gratitude.

2. Empathetic Communication: Practice active listening, empathy, and compassion in your interactions with others. Strive to understand different perspectives and foster mutual respect and understanding.

Lifestyle Choices

1. Holistic Self-Care: Prioritize self-care practices that nurture your body, mind, and spirit. This may include activities such as massage, aromatherapy, mindfulness walks, or creative expression.

2. Environmental Consciousness: Adopt eco-friendly habits and contribute to environmental sustainability. Reduce waste, conserve resources, and cultivate a deeper appreciation for the interconnectedness of all life.

Lifelong Learning

1. Continuous Growth: Embrace a growth mindset and a commitment to lifelong learning. Seek out opportunities for personal and professional development that align with your values and interests.

2. Exploration of Holistic Modalities: Explore holistic modalities such as acupuncture, herbal medicine, energy healing, or traditional practices from various cultures. Keep an open mind and integrate what resonates with you into your wellness journey.

CHAPTER SIX

DELICIOUS RECIPES IDEAS FOR THE 4:3 INTERMITTENT FASTING DIET

DELICIOUS 4:3 DIET BREAKFAST RECIPES

Bloody Mary Smoothie

Ingredients

• 3 medium tomatoes, chopped

• 2 tablespoons tomato paste

• 1/2 cup (66g) celery, diced (about 2 ribs)

• 1/2 medium avocado, pitted and peeled

• 1 tablespoon fresh horseradish, minced (not horseradish sauce), plus more to taste

• 2 1/2 teaspoons Worcestershire sauce, plus more to taste

• 10 dashes Tabasco sauce, plus more to taste

• 2 1/2 tablespoons freshly squeezed lemon juice, plus more to taste

• 1 teaspoon red onion, finely chopped

• 1 clove garlic, peeled

• 1 teaspoon natural salt

• Pinch freshly ground black pepper, plus more to taste

• 2 cups (250g) ice cubes

Optional boosters:

• 2 teaspoons cold-pressed extra virgin olive oil

• 1 teaspoon chia seeds

• 1 teaspoon goji powder

Preparation

1. Blend all **Ingredients** together:

Throw all of the **Ingredients** into the blender and blast on high for about 1 minute, until smooth and creamy. Tweak flavors to taste (you may want more horseradish, Worcestershire, Tabasco, lemon juice, or pepper).

Holiday Spice Granola

Ingredients

• 1/2 cup maple syrup

• 1/3 cup coconut oil

• 1 tablespoon vanilla extract

• 1 teaspoon ground cinnamon

• 1 teaspoon ground ginger

• 1/2 teaspoon salt

• 1/4 teaspoon ground cloves

• 5 cups old-fashioned rolled oats (not instant; use gluten-free oats, if needed)

- 2/3 cup flax seeds

- 2/3 cup pumpkin seeds

- 1/2 cup whole almonds

- 1/2 cup cashews

- 1/3 cup chia seeds

- 1 /2 cup dried cranberries

- 1/2 cup diced dried apricots

Preparation

1. Heat the oven to 350F:

Line a rimmed baking sheet with a piece of parchment paper that is about 1 inch larger all around than the baking sheet.

2. Make the syrup:

In a saucepan over medium heat, stir together the maple syrup, coconut oil, vanilla, cinnamon, ginger, salt, and cloves. Stirring occasionally, cook for 2 minutes, or until the syrup is warm and fluid, and the salt dissolves.

Mix the granola:

In a large bowl, combine the oats, flax seeds, pumpkin seeds, almonds, cashews, and chia seeds. Pour the warm syrup over the nuts and grains. Stir to coat them thoroughly. Spread evenly on the baking sheet.

1. Bake the granola:

Bake for 15 minutes, then remove the pan from the oven. Grasp the corners of the parchment paper and pull them toward the center to mound the granola in a pile. Stir with a large spoon and spread the granola out again in one layer.

Return to the oven for 5 minutes. Remove and mound the granola in the center again. If it still looks pale in places, give it another stir, spread it back out, and return the pan to the oven to toast for 3 or 4 minutes more. (Total baking time is 20 to 25 minutes.) Leave on the baking sheet to cool completely.

2. Add fruit and store the granola:

Scatter the cranberries and apricots over the cooled granola and stir to combine. Transfer the granola to an airtight jar or tin, and store at room temperature for several weeks.

Frittata with Potatoes, Red Peppers, and Spinach

Ingredients

• 6 large eggs

• 1/4 cup (60ml) milk

• 2 1/2 tablespoons olive oil

• 3/4 teaspoon ground turmeric

• 1/2 cup diced red onions

• 2 cloves garlic, minced

• 8 ounces (225g) fingerling potatoes, thinly sliced down their length

• 1 medium red pepper, seeded and diced

• 1 scallion, thinly sliced

• 1 cup baby spinach

• Freshly ground black pepper

Preparation

1. Preheat oven to 400°F

2. In a small bowl, whisk eggs and milk together

Set aside.

3. Cook the onions and garlic:

Heat olive oil in a 10-inch oven-safe skillet or pan over medium heat. Add the turmeric and stir so that turmeric dissolves into the oil.

Add diced onions and cook, stirring occasionally, until they start to soften, about 2 minutes. Add minced garlic and stir for 30 seconds.

Cook the potatoes and other vegetables:

Add the potatoes and a generous pinch of salt and cook, stirring occasionally, until some of the slices start to brown, 5 to 6 minutes.

Add the red pepper and cook until they start to soften, about 2 minutes. Add scallions and spinach leaves and cook until the leaves start to wilt, stirring occasionally.

Pour egg mixture into the skillet

and reduce heat to medium-low. Cook until the eggs start to set on the bottom, about 2 to 3 minutes.

Place skillet in the oven and bake for 8 to 9 minutes, until the center is set

Remove skillet from oven with oven mitts. Let frittata cool for 5 minutes before serving. Cut into wedges and season with more salt and some ground pepper, if desired.

Frittata will keep refrigerated for 5 days. Leftovers can be eaten chilled or briefly warmed in the microwave.

Parfait with Maple Yogurt, Citrus and Pomegranate

Ingredients

• 2 cups (16 ounces) thick, plain Greek or Icelandic-style yogurt

• 1/4 cup (2 3/4 ounces) maple syrup

• 1/2 teaspoon ground cinnamon

• 1/4 teaspoon ground ginger

• 1/4 teaspoon ground cloves

• Pinch salt

• 5 navel oranges (about 7 1/2 ounces each)

• 4 pink grapefruit (about 8 ounces each)

• 1/2 cup (3 ounces) shelled pistachios, roughly chopped, plus more for garnish

• 1/2 cup (3 ounces) pomegranate seeds

Preparation

1. Make the yogurt:

In a mixing bowl, whisk together the yogurt, maple syrup, cinnamon, ginger, cloves, and salt until combined. Refrigerate for 1 hour.

Segment the citrus:

Using a sharp knife, trim the pole ends oranges so they lay flat on the cutting board. Follow the curve of the orange with your knife to remove the peel and pith, exposing the segments beneath. (If you miss any bits of peel or pith on your first round, do a second pass.)

Working over a bowl to catch the juices, cut between each membrane to remove the segments. Transfer the segments to a bowl and refrigerate until ready to assemble the parfaits. Repeat with the pink grapefruit. For better control when it comes time to assemble the parfaits, store each citrus separately.

(Don't discard the juice you collect while segmenting the citrus; set it aside for another use – whisk it into your favorite vinaigrette, mix it with mineral water for a refreshing beverage, or simply drink it straight.)

1. Toast the nuts:

In a small skillet over medium-low heat, toast the pistachios until they begin to smell rich and nutty, 1 to 2 minutes. Shake the skillet regularly to keep the nuts from scorching. Set aside to cool.

2. Strain the citrus:

Strain the citrus segments to remove any accumulated juices (this helps prevent the parfaits from getting runny).

3. Assemble the parfaits:

Into 4 stemless wine glasses or parfait glasses, spoon 1/4 cup of the yogurt mixture. Evenly distribute the citrus segments among the glasses, leaving enough of each for a second layer. Top each with 1 tablespoon pistachios and 1 tablespoon pomegranate seeds.

Repeat the layers once more, starting with the yogurt and ending with the pomegranate seeds. Garnish each parfait by scattering a few more pistachios over the top.

Serve:

Enjoy these parfaits cold and within two hours of being assembled.

Tuscan Scrambled Eggs

Ingredients

- 3 tablespoons extra virgin olive oil

- 1 large yellow onion, peeled and chopped

• 1 1/4 pound (600g) plum tomatoes, peeled and chopped or one 14-ounce can of diced tomatoes

• 6 eggs

• Salt and freshly ground pepper

Preparation

1. Cook the onions until golden:

Heat olive oil on medium heat in a nonstick skillet. Add the onions and cook until translucent, just starting to turn golden in color, about 6 minutes.

2. Add tomatoes, cook low and slow:

Add the tomatoes and cook over low heat until the liquid evaporates, about 40 minutes.

3. Add eggs:

Whisk the eggs in a bowl until well blended. Season with a little salt and pepper. Add the eggs to the tomato and cook over medium heat, stirring constantly, and scraping from the bottom with a wooden spoon.

Remove from heat as soon as the eggs begin to set, but are still moist, about 3 minutes. Turn out onto a serving plate. Serve immediately.

Oatmeal Buttermilk Pancakes

Ingredients

• 3 cups old-fashioned rolled oats

• 1/2 teaspoon baking powder

• 1/2 teaspoon baking soda

- 1/2 teaspoon ground cinnamon (optional)

- 1/4 teaspoon salt

- 2 large eggs

- 1 1/2 to 2 cups buttermilk

- 2 tablespoons vegetable oil or melted butter

- 2 tablespoons honey

- 1 teaspoon vanilla extract

- Vegetable oil (for the skillet)

Preparation

1. Grind the oats:

Set aside 1/2 cup of the oats to add to the batter later. In a food processor, grind the remaining 2 1/2 cups oats until the mixture resembles coarse whole-wheat flour, with a few particles of oats.

Make the batter:

Add the baking powder, baking soda, cinnamon, salt, eggs, 1 1/2 cups of the buttermilk, oil or melted butter, honey, and vanilla to the food processor bowl and pulse a few times, until blended.

Pour the batter into a bowl and stir in the remaining 1/2 cup oats. Let stand for 5 to 10 minutes. The mixture will not be not completely smooth, and it will thicken as it sits. If the batter becomes too thick at any point feel free to thin with some of the remaining buttermilk.

1. Heat a skillet or griddle:

Pour a few drops of oil into the skillet or griddle and spread with a paper towel. Set the pan over medium heat. The pan is hot enough when you drop a few drops of water on it and they sizzle. Turn the heat to medium-low.

2. Cook the pancakes:

Ladle about 1/3 cup of batter for each pancake onto the skillet. With the back of the ladle, spread the batter into 4-inch circles. Cook for 2 to 3 minutes, or until bubbles form on top and the bottoms look brown when you peek under the pancakes with a spatula. Turn them and cook for another 2 minutes, or until browned. Repeat until all the batter is used.

Serve the pancakes:

Serve them hot off the griddle or keep them warm in a 325°F oven on a wire rack set over a baking sheet. Serve with lots of butter, fresh fruit (if you wish), and maple syrup.

Buckwheat Waffles

Ingredients

- 1 1/2 cups buckwheat flour

- 2 teaspoons baking powder

- 1 teaspoon baking soda

- Pinch kosher salt

- Pinch cinnamon

- 2 large eggs, separated

- 2 large egg whites, for extra lightness

- 2 tablespoons sugar

- 1 cup milk

- 1/4 cup water

- 1 cup plain yogurt

- 1/2 cup (1 stick) butter, melted

- Extra pats butter, for serving

- Heated maple syrup, for serving

- Berries, for serving

Preparation

1. Preheat the waffle maker:

Turn on your waffle maker and set to medium.

2. Whisk the dry **Ingredients**:

In a large bowl, whisk together the buckwheat flour, baking powder, baking soda, salt, and cinnamon.

Beat the egg whites and sprinkle in sugar:

Place the egg whites in a medium bowl and beat with a hand mixer or egg beater. Sprinkle in the sugar as you beat the egg whites. Beat egg whites until you have soft peaks.

1. Whisk together the wet **Ingredients** :

In a medium bowl, whisk together the egg yolks, melted butter, yogurt, milk, and water.

2. Combine the wet and dry **Ingredients**:

Pour the yogurt mixture into the buckwheat flour mixture and stir until just combined. It's okay if it's a little lumpy.

Fold in the egg whites:

Stir a third of the beaten egg whites into the batter until completely incorporated. Gently fold the remaining beaten egg whites into the batter until just combined and there are no streaks of egg whites. Be gentle so that you do not deflate the egg whites too much.

Make the waffles:

Working in batches, pour or spoon the batter into the wells of the preheated waffle maker, until the batter almost come to the edges. You will know if you've over-filled it because the batter will spill out of the waffle maker. No harm done, but it's a little messy.

Cook until the waffle maker indicator indicates that the waffles are ready, or wait until steam stops rising out of the waffle maker. Gently pull the waffles out with a fork.

Serve:

Serve with pats of butter, warmed maple syrup, and fresh berries.

Easy Breakfast Casserole With Prosciutto

Ingredients

• 1 tablespoon extra-virgin olive oil

• 1 medium yellow onion, chopped

• 2 big handfuls tender greens, such as arugula, dandelion greens, baby kale, or spinach (tough stems removed)

• 1 1/2 cups asparagus, cut into 3/4-inch pieces

• 1 teaspoon kosher salt, divided

• 3 ounces thinly sliced prosciutto

• 2 packed cups cubed crusty bread, such as levain, baguette, or Italian bread (slightly stale is ok)

• 8 large eggs

• 1 cup low fat cottage cheese

• 1 cup 2% milk (or whatever kind you have in the fridge)

• Freshly ground black pepper

• 1 1/2 cups (3 oz) grated cheddar, divided

Preparation

1. Preheat the oven to 350°F

2. Sauté the vegetables:

Add oil to a 12-inch ovenproof skillet set over medium heat. I use cast iron, but any ovenproof skillet will do.

Add the onion and sauté until tender, about 5 minutes. Add the greens, asparagus, and 1/2 teaspoon salt and sauté until the greens wilt, about 2 minutes. Remove from heat.

Add the prosciutto and bread:

Tear the prosciutto slices into smaller pieces and distribute over the vegetables. Add the bread and stir everything together. Leave that to cool while you whisk the eggs.

Whisk the eggs:

In a large bowl, whisk together the eggs, cottage cheese, milk, the remaining 3/4 teaspoon salt, and several generous grinds of black pepper. Add 1/2 cup of the cheese and stir again. Pour the eggs over the vegetables and scatter the remaining cheese on top.

1. Bake the casserole:

Place the casserole in the oven and bake until it is just set with no obvious liquid remaining, about 35 minutes. It should be a little jiggly. Keep in mind that it will continue to cook a bit once it's out of the oven.

2. Serve:

Cool for 10 minutes. Cut into wedges and serve.

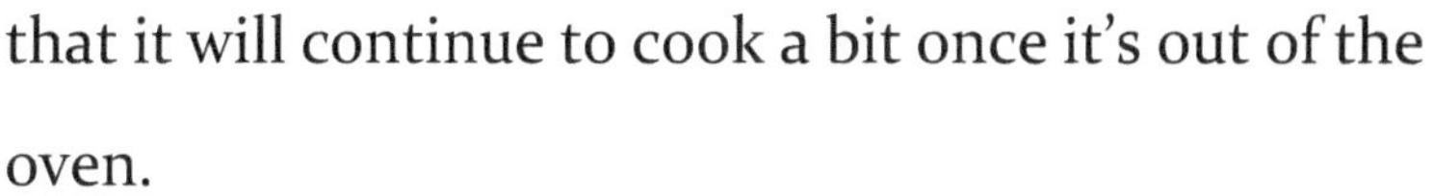

Orange-Spiced Whole Wheat Muffins

Ingredients

- For the muffin topping:

- 1/4 cup chopped walnuts

- 1/4 cup granulated sugar

- 1 teaspoon cinnamon

- For the muffins:

- 1 1/2 cup (195g) whole wheat pastry flour

- 1 cup (130g) all-purpose flour

- 1 1/2 teaspoons baking powder

- 1/2 teaspoon baking soda

- 3/4 cup (164g) granulated sugar

- 1/4 teaspoon kosher salt

- 2 teaspoons cinnamon

- 3/4 teaspoon ground cloves

- 3/4 teaspoon ground ginger

- 1/4 teaspoon nutmeg

• 2 teaspoons orange zest (from about 1 large orange)

• 2 large eggs, beaten

• 1 1/4 cups buttermilk

• 1/4 cup applesauce

• 5 tablespoons butter, melted

• 1 teaspoons vanilla extract

• 3/4 cup chopped walnuts

Preparation

1. Prep the pans and oven:

Line a muffin tin with cupcake liners. Preheat oven to 400°F.

2. Make the muffin topping:

In a small bowl, combine 1/4 walnuts, 1/4 cup granulated sugar, and 1 teaspoon cinnamon. Set aside.

Combine the flours and spices:

In a large bowl, whisk together whole wheat pastry flour, all-purpose flour, baking powder, baking soda, granulated sugar, salt, cinnamon, cloves, ground ginger, nutmeg, and orange zest.

Make the batter:

In a small bowl, whisk together eggs, buttermilk, applesauce, melted butter, and vanilla extract. Add the wet **Ingredients** to the dry **Ingredients** and stir to combine. The batter should be mostly combined with a few streaks of flour.

Add 3/4 cup walnuts, stir until incorporated. Do not overmix the batter; it will result in dense muffins.

Fill the muffin cups:

Fill muffin cups to the top with batter—don't worry, this is exactly how full you want them. Sprinkle with walnut and cinnamon sugar topping.

Bake the muffins:

Bake for 18 minutes until the muffins have crested over the pan and a toothpick inserted in the center comes out clean. They may show a combination of loose sugar and melted sugar.

The muffins should release from the just fine, but they may touch in a few places on the sides. Not to worry. Just use a knife to cut them apart before lifting them out of the pan. If the muffins are difficult to release from the pan, run a knife horizontally between the muffin top and the top of the muffin pan, taking care not to cut through the body of the muffin.

Serve warm with a pat of butter and a drizzle of honey. Or just eat them. Either way.

Store in an airtight container on the countertop for up to five days or freeze in a zip-top plastic bag. They will keep in the freezer for up to three months.

Microwave Oatmeal

Ingredients

• 1/4 cup steel-cut oats or old-fashioned rolled oats (not instant oats; use gluten-free oats if needed)

• 1/2 to 3/4 cup water, non-dairy milk, or milk

• Pinch salt

To serve — choose a few!

• Brown sugar, maple syrup, honey, or other sweetener

• Dried fruit, like dried cherries, cranberries, or figs

• Fresh fruit, like raspberries, blue berries, bananas, apples, or pears

• Chopped nuts, like pecans, pistachios, walnuts, or almonds

• Splash of milk, creme fraiche, or yogurt

Preparation

1. Combine the oats, water, and salt in a jar:

Use 1/2 cup of water for thick, spoonable oatmeal, or 3/4 cup for a softer, more porridge-like oatmeal. (You can also stir in additional liquid later on to thin it out, so no need to add too much here.) Secure the lid and swirl the contents a few times so that the oats are soaked.

Pack up your toppings:

Combine a handful of chosen oatmeal toppings in a small container. (If you're making multiple servings for breakfasts during the week, wait to assemble the toppings until the night before you plan to eat the oatmeal.)

1. Refrigerate overnight or up to 5 days.

2. Microwave the oatmeal:

Remove the lid from the container and set aside. If desired, transfer the oats and their soaking liquid to a separate microwave-safe bowl. Place the container on a microwave-safe plate (to catch any accidental spills), and place in the microwave.

Microwave on high power for 30 seconds, then remove the oatmeal and stir. Microwave for another 30 seconds, then remove and stir again. If the liquid is not quite piping hot, microwave for another 15 to 30 seconds, or as needed until the liquid is very hot. Cooking time may vary from microwave to microwave; in my microwave, 1 minute and 20 seconds total cooking time was perfect.

Microwave Poached Egg

Ingredients

• 1 large egg, straight from the refrigerator (see recipe note)

• 1/4 cup water

• Salt and pepper, for serving

Preparation

1. Microwave the water:

Put 1/4 cup water in an 8-ounce glass measuring cup or sturdy, microwave-safe mug.

Microwave on high power for 30 seconds to 1 minute, until the water is steaming (not rapidly boiling).

2. Add the egg, pierce the yolk, and cover:

Crack the egg into the water. Gently slide a toothpick into the yolk, keeping it intact. Cover the measuring cup or mug with plastic wrap (if using a mug, you may use a small microwave-safe saucer instead).

DELICIOUS 4:3 DIET LUNCH RECIPES

Fresh Salmon Salad

Ingredients

For the salmon:

• 1 pound salmon fillet, cut in half

• 1/2 teaspoon sea salt, for the rub

• 4 cups water

• 1 1/2 teaspoons sea salt, for the poaching liquid

• 1 slice lemon

• 1 teaspoon lemon juice

• 1 teaspoon extra virgin olive oil

For the salad:

- 2 stalks celery, finely chopped

- 1/2 red onion, peeled, finely sliced

- 1 tablespoon capers, strain out the pickling juice

- 1 teaspoon lemon zest

- 3 tablespoons lemon juice

- 1 tablespoon extra virgin olive oil

- 2 tablespoons fresh dill, chopped

- 1/8 teaspoon freshly ground black pepper

Preparation

1. Prep the salmon fillets:

Rub the salmon fillets all over with 1/2 teaspoon salt. Chill for 30 minutes in the refrigerator while you prep the other **Ingredients**.

2. Make the dressing:

Combine celery, red onion, capers, lemon zest and juice, dill, olive oil, black pepper in a large bowl. Set aside for the flavors to blend.

3. Poach the salmon:

Put 4 cups water, 1 1/2 teaspoons salt, and a slice of lemon in a pot wide enough to hold the salmon. Bring to a boil and simmer for about 5 minutes. Add the salmon to the pot. Return to a simmer and cook for 4 minutes at a bare simmer.

4. Cool and break up the salmon:

When the salmon is just cooked through, remove it from poaching liquid and put it in a bowl. Drizzle with a teaspoon of olive oil and a teaspoon of lemon juice. Once it has cooled to touch, break the salmon gently into chunks.

5. Make the salad:

Add the salmon to the bowl with the celery, onions, and capers. Gently toss to combine. Serve as is, or over mixed greens or butter lettuce.

Black Rice Bowls with Tofu and Veggies

Ingredients

For the miso ginger salad dressing:

• 1 piece (1-inch) fresh ginger, peeled and thinly sliced

• 1/2 clove garlic, thinly sliced

• 1/4 cup water

• 2 tablespoons rice vinegar

• 2 tablespoons red miso (See recipe note)

• 1 tablespoon low-sodium soy sauce

• 1 tablespoon honey

• 1/4 cup olive oil

• 1 tablespoon toasted sesame oil

For the baked tofu:

- 14 ounces (1 block) extra-firm tofu

- Olive oil spray

- 3 scallions, white and light green parts, thinly sliced

For the rice:

- 1 cup black rice or forbidden rice

- 6 cups water

- 1 teaspoon kosher salt

For the pickles:

- 1 cup unseasoned rice vinegar

- 3 teaspoons salt, divided

• 2 tablespoons sugar

• 1/2 cup water

• 1/2 small head cauliflower, cut into small florets

• 3 Persian (small) cucumbers

• 1 tablespoon low-sodium soy sauce

• 1 teaspoon sesame oil

For the kale:

• 1 bunch kale (any kind), washed, dried and stems removed

• 2 tablespoons olive oil

• Kosher salt to taste

To serve:

• Toasted almonds, for garnish

• Cilantro leaves or Thai basil, for garnish

• 1/4 cup currants, for garnish

Preparation

1. Make the salad dressing:

In a blender, finely chop the ginger and garlic.

Add the water, vinegar, miso, soy sauce, honey, olive oil and sesame oil and blend until smooth. (Dressing will keep for at least a week in the refrigerator.)

1. Preheat the oven: Preheat the oven to 475°F. Coat a baking dish or baking sheet with nonstick cooking spray.

2. Coat the tofu with miso, bake, then toss with more miso and scallions:

Cut the tofu into 1-inch cubes and thoroughly pat dry with paper towels.

Place the tofu in a bowl and add 3 tablespoons of the miso dressing. Toss to coat and transfer to the baking dish. Bake for 25 to 30 minutes, or until golden brown. Toss with the scallions and an additional 2 tablespoons of the miso dressing. Set aside.

The tofu can be baked up to three days ahead; wait to toss with scallions and the additional miso dressing until ready to serve.

Salmon Avocado Poke Bowl

Ingredients

For the poke bowl

- 1 cup short-grain white rice

- 1 pound sashimi-grade salmon

- 1/4 cup soy sauce

- 1 1/2 tablespoons rice vinegar

- 1/2 tablespoon sugar

- 1 teaspoon toasted sesame oil

- 1/4 teaspoon garlic powder

• 2 scallions, thinly sliced

Other toppings

• Sliced cucumber

• Sliced radish

• 1 large avocado, cubed

• Furikake

• Red pepper flakes

Preparation

1. Cook the rice:

Start the rice first and prep the rest of the **Ingredients** while it cooks. Rinse the rice a few times under cool water, rubbing it gently with your hands, until the water isn't quite so cloudy. Then cook the rice according to package instructions or in a rice cooker. Fluff and keep covered until ready to eat.

2. Prepare the salmon:

Gently pat the salmon all over to make sure that there are no pin bones still lodged in the fillet; if there are, use needle-nosed pliers to remove them. Cut the salmon into 1/2-inch cubes. Add the salmon into a medium bowl and set aside.

1. Make the dressing:

In a small bowl, stir together the soy sauce, rice vinegar, sesame oil, sugar and garlic powder. The garlic powder and sugar will not dissolve completely, but that's fine.

2. Combine the salmon and the dressing:

Add the sliced scallions to the bowl with the salmon, saving 1 to 2 tablespoons for garnish. Add the soy sauce mixture to the salmon and scallions. Using a large spoon or a rubber spatula, gently mix the salmon with the soy sauce mixture.

Serve:

Divide the rice between each bowl and then the salmon. Top with the rest of the sliced scallions, sliced cucumber, sliced radishes, diced avocado, furikake and red pepper flakes, if you like. The poke bowl is best enjoyed immediately.

Enfrijoladas with Black Beans, Avocado and Cotija

Ingredients

- 1 tablespoon extra virgin olive oil

- 1 large red onion, thinly sliced, divided

- 2 large cloves garlic, thinly sliced

- 1 chipotle chili in adobo sauce

- 2 (15-ounce) cans black bean, not drained or 3 1/2 cups cooked beans plus 1 cup bean cooking liquid

- 2 tablespoons lime juice

- 1/2 teaspoon ground cumin

- 1 teaspoon kosher salt

• 8 corn tortillas

• 2 small avocados, cut into slices

• 1/2 cup crumbled cotija cheese

• 1/3 cup Mexican salsa

• 1/3 cup light or regular sour cream

• 1/3 cup chopped cilantro

Special Equipment:

• Blender

Preparation

1. Sauté the onion and garlic:

Heat the olive oil in a large skillet over medium. Add 3/4 of the sliced onion and sauté until nearly tender, about 5 minutes. Add the garlic and sauté to soften, 2 minutes.

Blend the sauce:

Transfer the cooked onion and garlic to a blender along with the beans, including the bean liquid, chipotle, lime juice, cumin, salt, and 1/2 cup water. Blend until smooth and creamy. Taste and add more salt if needed, then blend again.

Heat the sauce:

Transfer the beans back to the large skillet set over low heat. Cook for 4 to 6 minutes at simmer. The sauce should be the texture of a thick soup. Add more water, if needed, to thin to the appropriate consistency.

Assemble the dish:

Use a pair of tongs to heat a tortilla over a gas flame or in a dry skillet set over high heat until it begins to blister. Submerge the tortilla in the bean sauce, smothering it completely. Use a spatula to fold it in half and transfer to a dinner plate. Top with a tablespoon of cotija, a slice or 2 of avocado, and a tangle of raw sliced onions. Continue with remaining tortillas and bean sauce, figuring 2 enfrijoladas per plate.

Serve:

Serve immediately with the salsa, cilantro, sour cream and any remaining bean sauce for guests to add as they please.

Shakshuka with Feta, Olives, and Peppers

Ingredients

• 2 tablespoons olive oil

• 1 teaspoon smoked paprika

• 1 teaspoon ground cumin

• 1/4 teaspoon Maras or Aleppo pepper flakes, or 1/8 teaspoon crushed red pepper flakes

• 1 large yellow onion, halved and thinly sliced

• 2 cloves garlic, thinly sliced

• 1 red bell pepper, seeded and thinly sliced

• 1 yellow bell pepper, seeded and thinly sliced

• 1 can (28 ounces) whole peeled tomatoes, preferably San Marzano

• 1/2 teaspoon salt, or to taste

• 4 ounces feta cheese, crumbled

• 1/3 cup pitted Kalamata or other olives in brine

• 4 large eggs

For garnish:

• 1/4 bunch cilantro, leaves coarsely chopped (for garnish)

Preparation

1. Cook the onion and peppers:

In a large skillet over medium heat, heat the oil. Add the paprika, cumin, and pepper flakes and cook for 30 seconds to a minute to bloom the spices.

Add the onion and cook, stirring occasionally, for 3 minutes. Add the garlic, red pepper, and yellow pepper and cook, stirring occasionally, for 15 minutes, or until the vegetables soften.

Crush the tomatoes and simmer them with the peppers:

In a bowl, break up the tomatoes with your hands. Add them to the skillet with the salt and cook for 5 minutes. Taste and add more salt, if you prefer.

Cook the eggs:

With the back of a spoon or a ladle, make 4 indentations in the sauce.

Break an egg into a cup and carefully pour it into and indentation, being careful not to break the yolk. Repeat with the remaining eggs. (You can crack the egg directly into the sauce and skip the cup, but it's easier to get a an errant egg shell or protect the dish from a bad egg if you use the cup Preparation.)

Sprinkle the feta and olives around the eggs. Cover the pan and simmer over medium heat for 8 minutes, or until the whites are set and the yolks are still soft. (If you like your eggs well done, cook for a minute or two longer.)

To serve:

Garnish with cilantro leaves and a sprinkling of red pepper flakes. Bring to the table and serve from the pan.

Easy Vegetable Tart with Carrots, Fennel and Chèvre

Ingredients

- 3/4 cup (100g) whole-wheat flour, spooned and leveled

- 3/4 cup (100g) all-purpose flour, spooned and leveled

- 1 teaspoon kosher salt, divided

- 8 tablespoons (122g) cold unsalted butter, cut into 16 or so little pieces

- 1/4 cup ice cold water

- 4 large carrots

• 1 medium/large bulb fennel

• 1 medium purple onion

• 1 1/2 tablespoons extra-virgin olive oil

• 1/4 teaspoon freshly ground black pepper

• 4 ounces soft herb goat cheese (chevre)

• 1 egg white

Preparation

1. Preheat and prep:

Preheat oven to 400°F and lay a 13x15-inch piece of parchment paper on your work surface. You will use it for the dough.

2. Prepare the dough:

Into a food processor fitted with the metal blade, add the whole-wheat flour, all-purpose flour, and 1/2 teaspoon Kosher salt. Scatter the cubed butter over the flour. Pulse the food processor until the **Ingredients** clump together like little peas. Add the water and run the food processor for several seconds (about 8 to 10) until the dough comes together in large clumps.

Shape the dough:

Dump the dough on the parchment paper and pat it into a smooth ball. Press the dough into a disk, scatter flour lightly over the top, and roll out the dough into a circle that's 13-inches in diameter (the width of the parchment paper). It doesn't need to be perfect.

1. Refrigerate the dough:

Transfer the dough to a baking sheet and refrigerate while you prep the vegetables.

2. Prep the vegetables:

Peel and trim the carrots and cut into 1/3-inch-thick coins. Cut the fennel in half, trim out the small triangle of core, and cut into 1/3-inch-thick wedges. Peel and slice the onion in half. Then slice into 1/4-inch-thick half moons.

3. Roast the vegetables:

Pile carrots, fennel, and red onion onto a large baking sheet and drizzle with the olive oil. Season with 1/2 teaspoon kosher salt and black pepper. Roast until tender, about 30 minutes.

Assemble Galette:

Set the baking sheet with the chilled dough on your work surface. Use a spoon to arrange the roasted vegetables in the center, leaving a 2-inch border. Crumble the goat cheese over the vegetables and use your fingers to nestle some of the cheese into the vegetables.

Form the dough:

Gently fold the edges of the dough over the vegetables, pleating and pinching it to stay in place (the center will stay exposed). Use a pastry brush to lightly coat the top of the galette with egg white.

Bake:

Bake in the oven for 40-45 minutes until nicely browned and crisp.

Enjoy:

Serve warm from the oven or room temperature. Cut into wedges and serve.

Crispy Baked Fish Sandwiches with Avocado Mayo and Pickled Onion

Ingredients

For the pickled onion

• 1/3 cup apple cider vinegar

• 1 tablespoon sugar

• 1 teaspoon kosher salt

• 1/2 medium red onion, thinly sliced

For the fish sandwiches

• 1 1/4 pounds firm white fish such as halibut, cod, or grouper

• 1 1/4 teaspoons kosher salt, divided

• 1/4 teaspoon ground black pepper

• 1 cup panko style breadcrumbs

• 1 tablespoon garlic powder

• 1 tablespoon ground cumin

• 2 large eggs

• 1/4 cup all-purpose flour

• Non-stick cooking spray

For the avocado mayo

- 1 large ripe avocado, peeled and pitted

- 1 tablespoon lime juice

- 2 tablespoons mayonnaise

To serve

- 4 soft sandwich buns, such as brioche

- 2 cups romaine hearts, shredded

- 2-3 tablespoons pickled jalapenos

Preparation

1. Preheat the oven, pickle the onions:

Preheat the oven to 425° F.

In a small shallow bowl, combine the vinegar, sugar, and 1 teaspoon salt and stir until the sugar and salt dissolve.

Submerge the onions in the liquid and set aside. Stir the onions occasionally, pressing them into the liquid, while you prep the sandwiches.

1. Sally Vargas

2. Cut and season the fish:

Cut the fish into 4 equal pieces that will work well with the bun size. Season all sides with 1 teaspoon kosher salt and black pepper.

1. Set up your workstations for the fish:

Generously coat a baking sheet (the darker the better) with cooking spray.

In a small shallow bowl, combine the panko, garlic powder, and cumin. In another small shallow bowl, crack and whisk the eggs. In a third shallow small bowl, add the flour.

Organize your workstation as such: flour, eggs, panko, baking sheet.

2. Dredge fish:

Dip a piece of fish in the flour to coat it on all sides, shaking off excess. Submerge the fish in the beaten eggs, coating all sides, and allow the excess to drip off. Finally, dredge fish in the seasoned panko until thoroughly coated on all sides. Lay on the sheet pan. Repeat with the remaining pieces of fish.

Coat fish with cooking spray and season:

Generously coat the top of the fish with non-stick cooking spray as if adding a coat of paint. Sprinkle with a pinch of kosher salt over the top of each piece of fish.

Bake fish:

Bake the fish on the top rack of the oven, until nicely browned on the underside, and just cooked through (it should flake when you pry it in the center with a fork), 10 to 12 minutes depending on thickness of the fish.

Make avocado mayo:

While the fish bakes, mash avocado in a small bowl using a fork. Add the lime juice, mayonnaise, and remaining 1/4 teaspoon kosher salt and combine until fairly smooth.

1. Warm buns in oven:

Place the buns on a baking sheet and put them in the oven to warm, about 1 minute. You want the buns soft and warm, not fully toasted.

2. Assemble fish sandwiches:

To assemble, spread avocado mayo on the bottom and top of the buns, top with the lettuce and followed by a piece of fish. Top the fish with a tangle of pickled onions and as many pickled jalapenos as you desire. Cover with the top bun. Serve

Spring Vegetable Salad with Asparagus, Peas and Radishes

Ingredients

For the salad:

• 1 teaspoon extra virgin olive oil

• 1/4 heaping cup sliced almonds

• 1/8 teaspoon salt, plus more for seasoning the salad

• 1/2 cup fresh or frozen (defrosted) English peas

• 6 stalks asparagus, tough ends trimmed

• 15 snap peas, strings stripped off

• 4 radishes

• 1 head butter lettuce, washed and torn into large pieces

• 1/4 cup loosely packed fresh mint (or fresh dill, tarragon or a combination), roughly chopped

• Freshly ground black pepper

For the dressing:

• 2 tablespoons crème fraîche

• 1/4 cup extra virgin olive oil

• 1 tablespoon fresh lemon juice

• Zest from 1/2 lemon

• 3 tablespoons fresh chives, minced

• 1 teaspoon Dijon mustard

• 1/2 teaspoon kosher salt

Preparation

1. Toast the almonds:

Heat 1 teaspoon olive oil in a medium skillet set over medium heat. Add the almonds and 1/8 teaspoon of salt and toast in the pan, stirring occasionally, until almonds are browned across the surface, about 5 minutes.

Transfer to a plate to cool.

1. Blanch peas if needed:

If using fresh or frozen peas that are sweet and tender, leave them as is and add into a large bowl.

If the peas are a bit starchy, blanch in a pot of salted boiling water until just tender, 2 to 3 minutes. Drain peas, and immerse in ice water, then drain and put in a large serving bowl. Set aside.

2. Cut veggies and assemble salad:

Cut the asparagus and snap peas on a diagonal into very thin slices. You should have about 1 cup of each. Cut the radishes into paper thin slices. Add the asparagus, snap peas, radishes, lettuce, and mint into the bowl with the peas.

Make the salad dressing:

Whisk together the crème fraîche, olive oil, lemon juice, lemon zest, chives, mustard, and salt in a small bowl.

Dress the salad:

Drizzle about two-thirds of the dressing over the salad, toss well. Add more dressing if needed and toss again (you may have some leftover dressing). Taste and season with fresh ground black pepper and salt, if needed. Garnish with toasted almonds. Serve immediately.

DELICIOUS 4:3 DIET DINNER RECIPES

Ginger-Soy Tilapia

Ingredients

• 3 tablespoons mirin

• 2 tablespoons water

• 2 tablespoons soy sauce

• 1 tablespoon rice wine vinegar

• 2 teaspoons minced ginger

• Cooking spray

• 3 frozen tilapia fillets, or other flaky white fish

• 1 teaspoon sesame oil

• 1 scallion, thinly sliced on the bias

• Sesame seeds, for garnish

Preparation

1. Put the cooking liquid in the pressure cooker:

Remove the lid to your Instant Pot. Into the Instant Pot add the mirin, water, soy sauce, vinegar, and ginger. Give it a quick stir.

Lightly grease a steamer rack with cooking spray and lower it into the Instant Pot insert as well. Set the frozen fillets on top of the steamer rack making sure to avoid overlapping the fish (if the fish overlap, they cook unevenly).

Lock on the lid and make sure the valve is set to seal.

1. Program the pressure cooker:

If your fish fillets are 1/2-inch thick or under, program the pressure cooker on the manual setting for 2 minutes at high pressure.

If your fish is thicker than 1/2-inch thick pieces, program your cooker on the manual setting for 3 minutes on high pressure.

The Instant Pot will take 6-7 minutes to come up to pressure before the actual cooking time begins.

2. Release the pressure, open the Instant Pot, and remove the fish:

Once the pressure-cooking time is up and the Instant Pot beeps, quick release the pressure using the steam vent. You can use the handle of a wooden spoon to release the pressure on the Instant Pot. Open the lid and lift the rack with the fish out.

The fish should be opaque and stained brown in patches from the steaming liquid. It won't be pretty, but don't worry about it.

To tell if the fillets are fully cooked through, prod the fish gently with your finger and it should easily flake apart. Cover loosely with foil to keep warm.

If the fish is not flaky after you quick release the pressure, add it to the liquid in the Instant Pot and cook it on the sauté setting until it's done.

Reduce the liquid to a glaze:

You can skip this step, but it makes for a tastier dish. Once you remove the fish, turn the sauté setting on high and boil the liquid until it's reduced by about half, enough to thicken and get sticky like a glaze, about 3 minutes.

Monitor the liquid all the while to make sure it does not burn. Stir in the sesame oil.

Garnish and serve:

Divide the fish between serving plates and pour the glaze over top. Garnish with a sprinkling of scallion greens and sesame seeds.

Parchment Baked Fish and Vegetables with Chermoula

Ingredients

• 3 tablespoons chermoula

- 1/2 cup bell pepper, thinly sliced

- 3/4 cup asparagus, cut into 2-inch pieces

- 3/4 cup zucchini, sliced in 1/4-inch-thick semi circles or coins

- 1/4 cup onion, cut into 1/8-inch-thick slices

- 2 (4-ounce) barramundi fish fillets

Preparation

1. Preheat the oven:

Preheat the oven to 425°F and make the chermoula recipe (It only takes a few minutes).

2. Make the parchment packets:

Cut off a piece of parchment about 16 inches long. Lay it down on a cookie sheet. Fold the paper in half lengthwise (short side to short side). Press the fold to make a crease, then reopen.

Place the **Ingredients** on the parchment paper:

Place the bell peppers, asparagus, zucchini, and onion on one half of the parchment paper. Leave enough room around the edges to fold the parchment together later. Add the fish on top of the vegetables and spread 3 tablespoons of chermoula all over.

Seal the fish and vegetables in parchment:

Fold the top piece of parchment over the fish and vegetables. You are going to fold, crease and press the top and the bottom pieces of parchment together to seal the food in the parchment.

Start at one end and fold the two pieces of parchment together pressing down to seal the folds while working your way around to the other side. Tuck your final fold underneath the parchment so the steam won't escape while the fish is baking. If you're finding it difficult to keep the parchment together you can staple it or use aluminum foil, especially if it's your first time doing this.

Though there is no twisting involved, the overall appearance will be slightly rolled or twisted looking.

1. Bake the fish:

Place the baking sheet with the parchment enrobed fish into the oven and bake the fish until it is feels fairly firm to the touch when you press on the outside of the parchment paper, about 15 minutes.

You should be able to press your thumb into the fish and your finger and be unable to push fully into it and create a dent; it should instead have a little bit of spring back. Remove from oven.

2. Let the fish rest and cool slightly:

Let the fish rest and cool slightly, about 5 minutes. The fish will continue to cook while it rests.

Once the fish has rested use scissors to slice through the parchment paper and transfer the fish and veggies onto a plate.

Note that hot steam will escape when opening the parchment packet—that's why it's imperative to let it cool for a few minutes, so that the steam doesn't burn you.

Mediterranean Chickpea Salad

Ingredients

For the vinaigrette

• 2 tablespoons olive oil

• 2 tablespoons red wine vinegar

• 1 teaspoon dried oregano

• 1/2 teaspoon kosher salt, plus more as needed

• 1/4 teaspoon freshly ground black pepper, plus more as needed

For the salad

• 2 (15-ounce) cans chickpeas, drained and rinsed

• 1 (12 ounce) jar quartered and marinated artichoke hearts, drained

• 1 pint cherry tomato or grape tomatoes, halved

• 2 Persian cucumbers, halved lengthwise and thinly sliced

• 2/3 cup pitted Kalamata olives, halved

• 4 scallions (about 1/2 cup), white and green parts, thinly sliced

• 2 tablespoons fresh mint leaves, chopped

• 6 ounces (about 1 1/2 cups), feta cheese, crumbled

Preparation

1. Make the oregano vinaigrette:

In a large bowl, whisk together the olive oil, red wine vinegar, dried oregano, kosher salt, and freshly ground black pepper.

Add salad **Ingredients** to vinaigrette:

Add the chickpeas, artichoke hearts, tomatoes, cucumbers, olives, scallions, and mint to the bowl. Toss well to combine and coat in the vinaigrette. Add the feta cheese and toss gently to combine. Taste and season with additional salt and pepper as needed.

Serve:

Serve immediately or cover and refrigerate. You can keep this salad in the fridge covered, for 5 days. Enjoy cold or at room temperature.

Baked Tilapia in Lemon Butter Sauce

Ingredients

• 1 1/2 pounds tilapia fillets

• 1/4 teaspoon kosher salt

• 1/8 teaspoon freshly ground black pepper

• 4 tablespoons unsalted butter

• 1 tablespoon garlic, minced

• 4 teaspoons lemon juice

Preparation

1. Preheat the oven and position rack:

Position a rack in the center of the oven. Preheat the oven to 450°F.

2. Pat fish dry and season:

Pat the fish dry using a paper towel. In a large baking dish, arrange the fillets in a single layer, making sure they do not overlap. Season the fillets with salt and pepper. Set aside.

Make the butter sauce:

In a small skillet over medium heat add the butter. Once the butter has melted add the garlic and cook until aromatic, about 2 minutes. Add the lemon juice and remove from the heat. Pour the sauce over the fish, trying to get the garlic bits on top of the fillets rather than the pan.

Bake the fish:

Bake the fish, until it is opaque and easily flakes apart when gently prodded, about 10 minutes. Serve immediately, spooning the sauce over the fish.

Herb Chicken Burgers

Ingredients

For the lemon mayo

- 1/2 cup mayonnaise

- 1 teaspoon lemon zest

- 1 tablespoon lemon juice

- 1/8 teaspoon salt

• 2 tablespoons fresh chives, finely chopped (optional)

For the chicken burger

• 1 pound ground chicken

• 1 large egg

• 1 cup breadcrumbs, divided

• 1 clove garlic, minced

• 1 teaspoon dried basil

• 1 teaspoon dried parsley

• 1/2 teaspoon kosher salt

• 1/2 teaspoon black pepper

To serve

* 4 brioche buns

* 1 ripe avocado, thinly sliced

* 1/2 red onion, sliced

* 1 medium tomato, sliced

Preparation

1. Make the lemon mayo:

In a small bowl, combine the mayonnaise, lemon zest, lemon juice, salt, and chives. Wrap the bowl in plastic wrap and set aside until you are ready to assemble your burgers.

2. Mix together chicken burger **Ingredients**:

In a medium bowl, combine the ground chicken, egg, ½ cup breadcrumbs, garlic, basil, parsley, salt, and pepper until thoroughly mixed.

To form patties, pour out the remaining 1/2 cup of breadcrumbs onto a plate.

Form the chicken patties:

Divide the chicken mixture into four even balls. Place one chicken ball at a time onto the plate of breadcrumbs.

Lightly press the chicken ball into the breadcrumbs on both sides to prevent it from sticking to your hands. Repeat until all the balls are coated.

Shape each ball into about a 1/2-inch patty and repeat with the remaining chicken balls until all of the burgers are formed.

1. Preheat the grill and add oil:

Preheat the grill for direct heat grilling, by turning gas burners to medium-high or spreading charcoal coals so there is direct heat under the grilling grates. The temperature should be 450-500°F.

To make sure the burgers do not stick, dip a clean kitchen towel or some paper towels in oil and use tongs to quickly rub down grill grates. Alternatively, you can spray the grates with spray oil, but be careful of flare-ups.

2. Grill the chicken burgers:

Grill the chicken burgers, about 4 minutes per side or until they reach at least 165°F in the center of the burgers using a thermometer.

Flip the burgers with a metal spatula, halfway through cooking, to help release any stuck burger pieces. The burgers will be done when they have excellent grill marks on both sides and are firm to pressure if you poke them.

Try not to overcook the burgers too much as they can dry ou

1. Grill the buns:

Grill the plain buns for 20 seconds and remove from the grill.

2. Assemble the burgers:

Add a few pieces of sliced avocado to the bottom bun. Top it with the grilled chicken burger, followed by sliced red onion, tomato slices, and a drizzle of the lemon mayo. Serve immediately.

Spicy Buffalo Chicken Burgers

Ingredients

For the burgers

• 1 pound ground chicken

• 1/2 cup panko breadcrumbs

• 2 tablespoons grated carrot

• 2 tablespoons grated celery

• 2 tablespoons Franks hot sauce, plus extra for serving

• 1/2 teaspoon kosher salt

• 1/2 teaspoon granulated garlic

• 1/4 teaspoon black pepper

To serve

• 4 potato hamburger buns

• Butter lettuce

• Blue Cheese Sauce

Preparation

1. Form the burgers:

In a large bowl combine the ground chicken, breadcrumbs, carrots, celery, hot sauce, salt, garlic, and black pepper. Shape mixture into four evenly-sized patties. They should be about 1/2-inch thick.

1. Preheat the grill and rub with oil:

Preheat the grill for direct heat grilling, by turning gas burners to medium-high or spreading charcoal coals so there is direct heat under the grilling grates. The temperature should be 450-500°F.

To make sure the burgers do not stick, dip a kitchen towel or some paper towels in oil and use tongs to quickly rub down grill grates. Alternatively, you can spray the grates with spray oil, but be careful of flare-ups.

2. Grilling the burgers:

Grill the buffalo chicken burgers, about 4-5 minutes per side or until they reach at least 165°F in the center of the burgers.

Chicken burgers are easy to overcook. The instant read thermometer really helps you find the sweet spot of fully cooked but still tender and juicy. Finished burgers will have grill marks on both sides and be firm to pressure.

1. Grill the buns:

Add buns to the grill next to burgers and grill for 30 seconds. Optionally, you can brush buns with a little butter or oil, but it isn't necessary.

2. Serve the burgers:

Serve the burgers on grilled potato buns with butter lettuce, blue cheese sauce, and an extra splash of Franks hot sauce.

Leftovers and storage:

Leftover buffalo chicken burgers keep well in the fridge for 3-4 days. They reheat really well in the microwave on high for 1 minute.

Lemon Chicken Soup (Avgolemono)

Ingredients

• 1 pound 2 ounces (500g) skinless chicken thighs on the bone

• 1/2 small white onion, finely chopped

• 2 fat cloves garlic, minced

• 1 small celery stalk, finely chopped

• 1 medium carrot, finely chopped

• 3/4 teaspoon ground cinnamon

• 1/4 teaspoon ground turmeric

• 2 bay leaves

• 3 1/4 cup (750ml) chicken stock

• 4 cups (960ml) just-boiled water, divided

• Scant 1/2 cup (90g) short or medium-grain white rice, rinsed

• 3 1/2 ounces (100g) kale, stalks removed, leaves shredded

• 3 extra large eggs

• 1 teaspoon finely grated unwaxed lemon zest

• 6 tablespoons lemon juice, or to taste

• 1 to 2 tablespoons chopped dill, or to taste

• Extra virgin olive oil

• Salt and black pepper

Preparation

1. Cook the chicken:

Place the chicken, onion, garlic, celery, carrot, cinnamon, turmeric, bay leaves, stock, and 2 cups (480 ml) hot water in a large saucepan. Season with 1 teaspoon salt and 1/2 teaspoon black pepper. Bring to a boil, then lower the heat, cover, and simmer for 40 minutes, until the chicken is cooked.

Remove and cool chicken, then shred and cook rice:

Spoon out the bay leaves and chicken and set aside on a plate to cool. Add the rice to the soup with remaining 2 cups (480ml) hot water. Cover and cook for 10 minutes. Meanwhile, use your hands to shred the chicken meat from the bones into very small pieces.

Cook kale and return chicken to pot:

After the rice has cooked, add the kale and return the chicken to the pot. Simmer for 5 minutes, then take off the heat.

Whisk eggs:

In a separate medium sized bowl, whisk together the eggs, lemon zest, and lemon juice until the mixture is foamy with no streaks remaining.

Temper the eggs:

Pour 2 ladles of broth from the saucepan into a cup. Then grab a whisk and slowly add this broth to the bowl of lemony eggs, a couple of tablespoons at a time, whisking constantly.

Don't pour in too much hot broth too quickly, or you'll end up with scrambled eggs. Increase to a steady stream once you are halfway through, still whisking, until you've incorporated all of it. Slowly drizzle the mixture back into the saucepan, whisking the soup constantly as you do so and incorporating it slowly.

Thicken soup:

Return the pot to low heat, add the dill, and cook for 5 minutes to allow the soup to thicken. Don't let it come up to more than a gentle simmer and, if it starts to look a bit too thick, simply loosen it with a bit of hot water.

Finish soup and serve:

Finally, taste and adjust the seasoning, adding a bit more lemon juice, herbs, salt, or black pepper to taste. Serve in warmed bowls with a drizzle of extra-virgin olive oil.

Plum and Peach Salad with Champagne Vinaigrette

Ingredients

For the salad

• 2 large eggs

• 2 slices bacon

• 3 lightly packed cups frisée, hand-torn into large pieces

• 1 ripe peach

• 2 ripe plums

For the vinaigrette

• 1 tablespoon champagne vinegar

• 2 tablespoons extra virgin olive oil

• 2 teaspoons Dijon mustard

• 1/4 teaspoon kosher salt

• 1/8 teaspoon freshly ground pepper

Preparation

1. Prepare the ice bath:

In a medium bowl, add 2 handfuls of ice, cover with water, and set aside. You will add the steamed eggs to the ice bath to stop the cooking process.

2. Steam the eggs:

To prepare a steamer basket: Fill a medium saucepan with about 1 inch of water. Set the steamer basket into the pot and bring the water to a boil over high heat.

To prepare using a saucepan: If you are not using a steamer basket, just fill the bottom of a saucepan with 1/2 inch of water. Bring water to a boil over high heat.

Turn off the heat and gently place the eggs at the bottom of the steamer basket or the bottom of the saucepan.

Turn the heat back on again to medium high and cover the pot. Steam the eggs for 6 1/2 to 7 minutes, for runny yolks. After they've steamed, transfer the eggs to the ice bath to cool and peel them right before you are ready to assemble the salad.

Cook the bacon:

Line a plate with a paper towel and set aside.

While the eggs are steaming, cook the bacon. In a medium pan over medium-high heat, cook the bacon slices until crisp, about 5 minutes, flipping halfway through. Transfer the bacon to the paper towel-lined plate.

Cut the stone fruit:

Cut the peach and plums into wedges: Cut the fruit in half and remove the pit, then cut into quarters or eights, depending on the size of the fruit.

If the pit clings to the fruit's flesh, you can cut one wedges while the flesh is still attached to the pit, cutting from the stem-end of the fruit down to the bottom, then pull the pieces away from the pit one by one.

Place the cut stone fruit into a medium mixing bowl.

Make the vinaigrette:

In a small jar with a lid combine the vinegar, olive oil, and Dijon mustard. Season with salt and pepper. Shake well to emulsify.

Prepare the frisée and dress the salad:

Tear the frisée into bite-sized pieces with your hands and add it to the bowl with the fruit. Start by drizzling half the dressing onto the frisée and fruit mixture, and gently toss to coat. Add more dressing, as needed, 1 tablespoon at a time, until well dressed.

Plate and serve salad:

Divide the frisée and fruit between two plates and crumble the bacon over top. Top each salad with one egg. Slice each egg in half so the yolk begins to run out onto the salad. Serve.

Zucchini Lasagna with Ground Turkey

Ingredients

• Non-stick cooking spray

• 5-6 medium (3 pounds) zucchini or yellow squash

• 3/4 teaspoon coarse kosher salt, divided

• 3/4 teaspoon freshly ground black pepper, divided

• 1 cup low-fat ricotta, optional

• 1 teaspoon pure olive oil

• 1 medium onion, chopped

• 4 garlic cloves, very finely chopped

• 1 pound ground turkey, preferably breast meat

• 1 (14.5 ounce) can crushed tomatoes

• 1 tablespoon chopped fresh basil

• 1 tablespoon fresh parsley, chopped, optional

• 1/4 teaspoon red pepper flakes, or to taste

• 1/3 cup shredded Parmesan cheese, divided

• 1 cup (4 ounces) shredded part-skim mozzarella cheese

Preparation

1. Preheat the oven and prepare baking dish:

Preheat the oven to 425°F. Spray an 8 by 8-inch baking dish with nonstick cooking spray. Set aside.

Line baking sheets and prepare squash:

Line 2 rimmed baking sheets with silicone mats or parchment paper. Remove the stem end of the squash. Slice the squash lengthwise into 1/4-inch thick strips.

Place the squash on the prepared baking sheets in a single layer. Season with 1/4 teaspoon salt and 1/4 teaspoon black pepper.

Cook squash:

Roast, rotating the baking sheets once halfway through cooking, until the squash is tender, about 25 minutes. Don't skip this step! The zucchini needs to be tender and cooked all the way through so it will not exude liquid into the lasagna.

Season the ricotta:

While the squash is roasting, place the ricotta it in a small bowl. Season with 1/4 teaspoon salt and 1/4 teaspoon black pepper. Stir to combine and set aside.

Cook the aromatics:

While the squash is roasting, set a large skillet over medium heat. Add the oil. Once the oil shimmers, add the onion and cook, stirring occasionally, until golden brown, 5 to 7 minutes. Add the garlic and cook until fragrant, 45 to 60 seconds

Make the meat sauce:

Add the turkey to the skillet with the onion and garlic. Season with the remaining 1/4 teaspoon salt and 1/4 teaspoon black pepper. Cook, breaking up the turkey with a wooden spoon until the turkey starts to cook on the outer edges, about 3 to 5 minutes.

Add the crushed tomatoes, basil, parsley, and red pepper flakes. Stir to combine and continue to cook until the meat is cooked through, and the mixture is fairly dry, and most of the moisture has evaporated, about 10 minutes.

Taste and adjust for seasoning with additional salt and pepper if needed.

1. Cool squash:

Remove the baking sheet of vegetables to a rack to cool slightly. You don't want them piping hot and falling apart. Leave the oven on. You will use it to bake the lasagna.

2. Assemble the lasagna:

Place 1 cup of the meat sauce in the bottom of the prepared baking dish. Place a single layer of squash strips on top, trimming all the squash strips to fit, if necessary.

Top with 1 cup of meat sauce, spreading with a spoon or spatula to lightly cover the vegetables. Sprinkle with 2 tablespoons of Parmesan cheese.

Add a second layer of squash strips perpendicular to how the first layer was placed. Top with 1 cup of meat sauce, spreading with a spoon or spatula to lightly cover the vegetables. Sprinkle with 2 tablespoons of Parmesan cheese.

Gently spread the ricotta over the squash and Parmesan using a spoon or spatula to help you. You'll be using all of the ricotta for this one layer.

Add a third layer of squash strips in the opposite direction of the last layer. Top with the final cup of meat sauce, spreading with a spoon or spatula to lightly cover the vegetables. (Your final lasagna will have 3 layers of squash and 4 layers of meat sauce including the top and bottom layers.)

Top with shredded mozzarella and sprinkle over the remaining tablespoon of Parmesan cheese.

Bake the lasagna then serve:

Transfer to the oven and cook until bubbly and golden brown, 25 to 30 minutes. Remove to a rack to cool slightly, then serve.

Lobster and Grilled Corn Panzanella

Ingredients

For the vinaigrette

- 1/4 cup white wine vinegar

- 1 clove garlic, minced

- 1 tablespoon fresh tarragon, finely chopped

- 2 teaspoons Dijon mustard

- 2 teaspoons kosher salt

- 1/8 teaspoon ground black pepper

- 1/2 cup extra virgin olive oil

For the salad

- 2 pints grape or cherry tomatoes, halved

- 1 small red onion, thinly sliced, divided

- 4 ears corn on the cob, unhusked

• 2 (8 ounce) frozen uncooked lobster tails, thawed and rinsed

• 5 (3/4-inch thick) slices Italian loaf or ciabatta

• 1 tablespoon extra virgin olive oil

• 1/4 teaspoon kosher salt, plus more to taste

• 4 Persian cucumbers, halved and cut crosswise into 1/2-inch pieces

• 1 teaspoon fresh tarragon, chopped

• 1 tablespoon fresh parsley, chopped

Preparation

1. Make the vinaigrette:

In a small mixing bowl, whisk together the vinegar, garlic, tarragon, mustard, salt and pepper.

Continue to whisk while slowly drizzling in the olive oil in a steady stream until the vinaigrette is emulsified.

2. Marinate the tomatoes and onions:

In a large wide shallow serving bowl, combine the tomatoes, half of the onions, and 1/2 cup of the vinaigrette. Set aside to let the tomatoes marinate and exude their juices as you prepare the rest of the salad.

Prep and soak the corn:

Peel off and remove the outermost layers of corn husk while keeping the majority of the husks still on the corn. Trim the corn silk tassels and tips of the husks hanging beyond the tip of the corn. Trim off the base of the corn so that it can stand flat when held upright. Only trim enough of the base so that the remaining husks don't fall off.

If your corn is very fresh, there's no need to soak them as they should still be very moist. If they're several days old, you may want to plump them up by soaking them in cold water for 20 to 30 minutes prior after preparing (as instructed above) to grilling.

1. Prepare the steamer basket:

In a pot large enough to hold the lobster tails in a single layer, add 1 to 2 inches of water so that a steamer basket isn't submerged. Add about 1 tablespoon of salt to the water.

Place the steamer basket into the pot. If you don't have a steamer basket, loosely scrunch some foil into balls and place them in the pot so they sit above the water level, giving the lobster tails a perch to rest on.

Cover the pot and bring the water to a boil over high heat.

2. Steam the lobster:

Place the lobster tails into the steamer basket, with the bottom side down, cover, and steam until the shells are red and the meat is opaque, about 10 minutes.

Transfer the lobsters to a shallow bowl or plate and let cool until you're able to handle with hands but still warm, about 5 minutes.

Remove lobster meat from shell:

Turn the lobster tail onto its back with the softer shell facing up. Using a pair of sharp scissors, cut along both edges of the soft shell from the wide end to the fan tail.

Grab the soft shell from the wide end and peel the soft shell off. Pull the meat out. Cut a long slit down top side of the tail meat. Use the tip of a small knife to remove the gray-black string of digestive vein if there is one.

Cut the lobster into bite-size pieces.

1. Prepare the grill:

Preheat the grill for high direct heat. You want it at 500°F.

2. Grill the bread:

Using a pastry brush, lightly brush both sides of the bread slices with oil and sprinkle with the salt. Arrange the bread in a single layer on clean grill grates and close the grill lid.

Grill the bread on both sides, until the bread has grill marks and is slightly toasty and slightly charred, 30 seconds to 1 minute per side. This is not the time to walk away as the bread can burn very quickly.

Remove the bread from the grill and set aside to let cool. Cut into 1/2-inch pieces.

Grill the corn:

Place the corn in a single layer on the grates, using long tongs if necessary. Close the lid and grill, turning the corn a couple of times to cook evenly, 8 to 10 minutes total.

Using tongs, remove one ear of corn from the grill and carefully peel back some of the husk to peek at the kernels. The kernels should have changed from a flat to shinier bright color. Remove all of the corn and set aside to let cool slightly, about 4 to 5 minutes.

One the corn is cool enough to handle, pull the remaining husk and silk off. It may help to grab the corn by the base with a kitchen towel if it's still hot and you want to get things rolling.

Return the corn to the grill, turning once or twice to get some smoky flavor and char on the kernels, 2 minutes. Don't grill them too long or they'll dry out. Remove corn from the grill and set aside to cool.

Cut corn kernels off the cob:

Working with one ear of corn at a time, hold the corn upright with the tip facing up in a wide shallow bowl. Using a sharp knife, I prefer a serrated one, cut downwards pressing the side of the knife against the cob as a guide, to separate the kernels from the cob.

Assemble the salad and serve:

Add the remaining onions, cucumbers, bread, lobster, and corn to the bowl of marinating tomatoes and onions and toss to coat evenly.

Sprinkle the tarragon and parsley over the salad and toss again. Season to taste with salt, if desired. Taste the salad and add additional vinaigrette as needed. Serve.

Grilled Oysters with Spicy Miso Butter

Ingredients

• 2 dozen medium to large fresh oysters in the shell

• 4 tablespoons unsalted butter, softened to room temperature

• 2 teaspoons white miso paste

• 1 1/2 teaspoons sriracha

• 1 large lime, zested

• 1 baguette, for serving

Preparation

1. Preheat your grill:

If you're using a gas grill, turn it to high, cover with the lid and let preheat for 10 minutes.

If using a charcoal grill, light the coals and let them get hot. The grill is hot enough when you hold your hand an inch above the grill grates and can only leave it there for a few seconds.

Make the miso butter:

In a small bowl combine the butter, miso paste, and sriracha using a fork until well blended. Set aside until ready to use.

Clean the oysters:

Rinse the oysters under cold running water. Use a scrub brush or kitchen towel to slough off any dirt.

Grill the oysters:

Place the oysters on the hot grill, flat-side up, and cover with the lid. Cook until the oysters crack open. They won't necessarily open wide like a clam, just look for a little crack.

Occasionally an oyster refuses to open. Not to worry, it will be fully cooked, and you can wedge it open using an oyster knife. If you open the oyster and it smells "off" or unpleasant, toss it out.

The time will vary depending on the heat of the grill and size of the oysters, 3 to 6 minutes.

Transfer to a platter and open oysters:

Use tongs to transfer the oysters to a platter, including any oysters that haven't cracked open (they are fully cooked and are fine to eat unless they have an unpleasant smell).

When the oysters are cool enough to handle, use an oyster or paring knife to pry the flat lid off each oyster and loosen it from the shell. Do your best not to spill the tasty oyster juices. You want each oyster tucked into the well of its shell. Discard the flat top shell.

Any oysters that haven't opened should be fairly easy to wedge open. Hold each unopened oyster using a sturdy kitchen towel to protect your hand and insert an oyster knife in the narrow end of the shell. Wiggle until the shell lifts off.

Spoon miso butter onto oysters and return to grill:

Spoon about 1/2 teaspoon of miso butter onto each oyster and set on the grill using tongs. Cover and grill until the butter bubbles, 30 to 60 seconds.

1. Transfer to a platter:

Spread uncooked rice or a rock salt over a large platter to help stabilize the oysters. (If you want to.) Place the oysters on top and add a little lime zest over the top.

2. Serve:

Serve with the baguette, to be torn and dunked into the melted miso butter that lingers in the shells.

Grilled Shrimp with Chermoula

Ingredients

For the chermoula

• 3 cloves garlic

• 2 cups cilantro, coarsely chopped

• 1 cup parsley, coarsely chopped

• 1 teaspoon finely chopped preserved lemon peel (optional)

• 1/2 teaspoon kosher salt

• 1/2 teaspoon ground cumin

• 1/4 teaspoon sweet paprika

• Pinch cayenne pepper

• 3/4 cup extra-virgin olive oil

• 2 tablespoons lemon juice

For the grilled shrimp

• 20 extra jumbo (16/20) shrimp, peeled and deveined, with tail on

• 1/2 teaspoon kosher salt

Preparation

1. Make the chermoula:

Pulse the garlic in a food processor until chopped. Add the cilantro, parsley, preserved lemon, if using, salt, cumin, paprika, and cayenne. Pulse until finely chopped. Add the oil and lemon juice and pulse until mixed.

The mixture will not be completely emulsified. The mixture will separate slightly with a layer of oil at the top and the slightly chunky mixture of herbs at the bottom.

1. Preheat the grill and soak the skewers:

If using wooden skewers add them to a wide shallow dish with water. Let them soak for 30 minutes. Preheat grill to medium-high direct heat. You want to bring it up to 450°F-500°F.

2. Marinate the shrimp:

In a wide shallow bowl or container, season the shrimp with salt and toss to coat in 3 tablespoons of the chermoula. Set aside to let marinate for 15 to 20 minutes. Reserve the rest of the chermoula sauce for serving.

Skewer the shrimp:

Thread the shrimp onto the soaked bamboo skewers through the top fatter section of the shrimp and through the section about 1/4-inch above the tail, adding five pieces of shrimp per skewer.

Grill the shrimp:

Using tongs, arrange the skewers of shrimp in a single layer on the grill. Grill shrimp until seared and slightly pink on the bottom side, 2 to 3 minutes. Flip, using tongs, and cook the other side until the shrimp is opaque, another 1 to 2 minutes.

Serve:

Using tongs, transfer the skewers to a platter. Let the shrimp cool slightly, then serve with the remaining chermoula on the side.

Cold Rice Noodle Salad

Ingredients

For the salad

- 14 ounces dried Dragonfly brand "rice sticks" or similar rice noodles

- 3 scallions, white and light green parts only

- 2 medium carrots

- 1 red bell pepper

- 1/2 English cucumber

- 2 cups (6 ounces) snow peas

- 1/2 cup cilantro leaves, roughly chopped

• Chinese chili oil or chili crisp, for drizzling

For the dressing

• 1 clove garlic, minced

• 1/4 cup light soy sauce

• 2 1/2 tablespoons Chinese black vinegar

• 1 tablespoon sugar

• 1/2 teaspoon sesame oil

Preparation

1. Cook the noodles:

Bring a large pot of water to a boil. Add the noodles and cook them until they are pliable but still fairly firm inside, about 6 minutes.

Turn off the heat, and let the noodles sit in the water until they are cooked through but still chewy, about 2 minutes. If you pull on a noodle, it should stretch quite a bit before it breaks.

Drain the noodles, and immediately rinse them in cold running water, massaging them gently to stop the cooking and to remove excess starch, until they are cool to the touch.

Meanwhile, prepare the vegetables:

Trim the roots off the scallions and cut them into 2- to 3-inch-long pieces. Cut them in half lengthwise, then slice them into very thin strips. Put them into a small bowl and cover them with cool water to let their flavor mellow a bit.

Peel the carrots and trim off the ends. Cut them into 2- to 3-inch-long pieces, then cut them into thin slices lengthwise, about 1/8-inch thick. This can be done with a mandoline. Cut the slices into thin strips.

Remove the stem and seeds from the bell pepper and slice it into long thin strips to match the carrots.

Cut the cucumber in half lengthwise. Use a spoon to scoop out the soft, seed-filled center and discard. Keep the skin on. Slice the cucumber lengthwise into thin strips matching the other vegetables.

Pinch off both ends of the snow peas and remove the string that runs along one side. Slice them lengthwise into thin strips.

Make the dressing:

In a small bowl, mix the garlic, soy sauce, vinegar, sugar, and sesame oil until the sugar dissolves.

Assemble and serve the salad:

Drain the scallions. In a large bowl, add the drained noodles, scallions, carrot, bell pepper, cucumber, and snow peas. Add the dressing and toss well to evenly coat. Top with the cilantro. Drizzle with the chili oil or serve it on the side.

Grilled Caprese-Stuffed Zucchini Boats

Ingredients

• 1 cup grape tomatoes, quartered

• 2 cloves garlic, finely minced

• 2/3 cup (3 ounces) fresh mozzarella cheese, cut into small cubes

• 1/4 cup freshly grated Parmesan cheese

• 2 teaspoons dried Italian seasoning

• 5 to 6 large fresh basil leaves, sliced into thin ribbons, plus 2 to 3 leaves for garnish

• 1/4 cup plus 1 tablespoon extra virgin olive oil, divided

• 1 teaspoon salt, divided

• 1/2 teaspoon freshly ground black pepper, divided

• 2 (8 to 10-inch) zucchinis

• 1 tablespoon balsamic vinegar, optional

Preparation

1. Preheat the grill:

If using a gas grill heat it to 350°F. If using a charcoal grill you want it hot enough so you can hold your hand a couple of inches above the grate for 4 to 5 seconds.

2. Make the caprese stuffing:

In a medium bowl, add the tomatoes, garlic, mozzarella, parmesan, Italian seasoning, basil, 1/4 cup of extra virgin olive oil, 1/2 teaspoon salt, and 1/4 teaspoon black pepper. Toss to combine and set aside to marinate while preparing the zucchini.

Prepare the zucchini for the grill:

Slice the zucchini in half lengthwise. Do not trim the ends. Use a metal spoon to scoop out the seeds. Brush the hollowed-out zucchini with the remaining 1 tablespoon of extra virgin olive oil. Season them with remaining 1/2 teaspoon salt and 1/4 teaspoon black pepper, if desired.

Grill the zucchini:

Place the zucchini halves cut side-down on the grill. Close the lid and cook for 5 to 10 minutes, checking them after 5 minutes, until browned and slightly softened. You do not want the zucchini to become too charred or overcooked.

Use tongs to transfer the zucchini onto a dish skin side-down.

Stuff the zucchini:

Fill each zucchini with the caprese stuffing.

Return the zucchini to the grill:

Using tongs transfer the stuffed zucchini back onto the grill, skin side-down. Close the lid and grill for 5 to 10 minutes, until the mozzarella is melted. Check for doneness after 5 minutes.

Serve warm:

Drizzle the zucchini boats with balsamic vinegar and sprinkle with additional fresh basil, if desired.

CHAPTER SEVEN

JUST ONE FINAL THING TO ADDRESS BEFORE YOU GO!

In conclusion, the 4:3 Diet presents a compelling approach to intermittent fasting, offering individuals a structured yet adaptable framework to optimize their health and well-being. Throughout this dietary regimen, the alternating cycle of four days of regular, balanced eating followed by three days of controlled fasting fosters a metabolic environment conducive to various health benefits.

While weight management is a primary focus, the 4:3 Diet extends its impact beyond mere physical outcomes, with proponents reporting improvements in metabolic health markers, cognitive function, and overall vitality.

What distinguishes the 4:3 Diet is its versatility and feasibility, accommodating diverse lifestyles and dietary preferences. Its inherent flexibility empowers individuals to tailor their fasting days to suit their unique needs, ensuring sustainability and long-term adherence. Moreover, the simplicity of the approach—eschewing complex meal plans or calorie counting—renders it accessible to a broad audience, from seasoned health enthusiasts to those new to dietary interventions.

Yet, success with the 4:3 Diet necessitates more than mere adherence to a prescribed eating schedule; it demands a holistic approach to health and wellness. Mindful eating practices, conscious food choices, and regular physical activity complement the fasting regimen, amplifying its efficacy and fostering a comprehensive approach to well-being. Additionally, cultivating a supportive environment, whether through social connections or professional guidance, can provide invaluable encouragement and accountability along the journey.

As individuals embark on their 4:3 Diet journey, it is essential to recognize the significance of self-awareness and self-compassion. Listening to one's body, respecting its signals, and honoring its needs are paramount, ensuring that the pursuit of health remains aligned with holistic principles. Furthermore, acknowledging that progress is nonlinear and embracing setbacks as opportunities for growth cultivates resilience and perseverance—a vital mindset for sustainable lifestyle changes.

Ultimately, the 4:3 Diet is not merely a temporary dietary intervention but a paradigm shift—a catalyst for transformative lifestyle changes rooted in self-care and self-improvement. By embracing its principles with intentionality and commitment, individuals can unlock their full potential for health, vitality, and longevity, embarking on a journey toward holistic well-being that extends far beyond the confines of a book's final page.

9 798327 066731